Understanding 6–7-Year-Olds

Corinne Aves

Jessica Kingsley Publishers
London and Philadelphia

First published in 2006
by Jessica Kingsley Publishers
116 Pentonville Road
London N1 9JB, UK
and
400 Market Street, Suite 400
Philadelphia, PA 19106, USA

www.jkp.com

Library of Congress Cataloging in Publication Data

Aves, Corinne.
    Understanding 6-7-year-olds / Corinne Aves ; foreword by Jonathan Bradley.
        p. cm. -- (Understanding your child series)
    Includes bibliographical references and index.
    ISBN-13: 978-1-84310-467-4 (pbk. : alk. paper)
    ISBN-10: 1-84310-467-9 (pbk. : alk. paper) 1. Child development. 2. Child psychology. 3. Children--Social conditions. I. Title. II. Title: Understanding six-seven-year-olds. III. Series.
    HQ767.9.A95 2006
    305.231--dc22

                                                        2006012328

British Library Cataloguing in Publication Data
A CIP catalogue record for this book is available from the British Library

ISBN-13: 978 1 84310 467 4
ISBN-10: 1 84310 467 9

Printed and bound in Great Britain by
Athenaeum Press, Gateshead, Tyne and Wear

Contents

Acknowledgements

With warm thanks to Annette Malin (and her class of 2005), Jo Cuttle and Peter Gordon at Hazelwood Infants School for generously sharing their work and thoughts. Many thanks, also, to all those who contributed to this book in direct and indirect ways, especially Margaret Rustin and Lisa Miller, the parents and children I have come to know, and my own six- and seven-year-olds, past and present.

Foreword

The Tavistock Clinic has an international reputation as a centre of excellence for training, clinical mental health work, research and scholarship. Established in 1920, its history is one of groundbreaking work. The original aim of the Clinic was to offer treatment which could be used as the basis of research into the social prevention and treatment of mental health problems, and to teach these emerging skills to other professionals. Later work turned towards the treatment of trauma, the understanding of conscious and unconscious processes in groups, as well as important and influential work in developmental psychology. Work in perinatal bereavement led to a new understanding within the medical profession of the experience of stillbirth, and of the development of new forms of support for mourning parents and families. The development in the 1950s and 1960s of a systemic model of psychotherapy, focusing on the interaction between children and parents and within families, has grown into the substantial body of theoretical knowledge and therapeutic techniques used in the Tavistock's training and research in family therapy.

The Understanding Your Child series has an important place in the history of the Tavistock Clinic. It has been issued in completely new form three times: in the 1960s, the 1990s, and in 2004. Each time the authors, drawing on their clinical background and specialist training, have set out to reflect on the extraordinary story of 'ordinary development' as it was observed and experienced at the time. Society changes, of course, and so has this series, as it attempts to make sense of everyday accounts of the ways in which a developing child interacts with his or her parents, carers and the wider world. But within this changing scene there has been something constant, and it is best described as a continuing enthusiasm for a view of development which recognizes the importance of the strong feelings and emotions experienced at each stage of development.

This book continues the complex story of development already unfolding in a dramatic way. The content of this individual volume will be made more meaningful when seen in the context of earlier volumes in the series. It has become clear that development is not only about looking forward, but also about connecting with the past. In a sense, then, 6–7-year-olds are still likely to return from time to time to an earlier version of themselves, but overall, as this volume shows, they are maturing over many fronts. The powerful image of the loss of milk teeth is set against the rapid development of coordination and balance, acquiring fine motor skills like drawing and writing, and generally amassing knowledge at a rapid pace. Inevitably the pace of such change can be too much to bear at times, and the book looks sensitively at the confusions and anxieties that can result from this. There is turmoil, inevitably, but within a process of maturing that sees the move away from infant school to the junior classes.

Jonathan Bradley
Child Psychotherapist
General Editor of the Understanding Your Child series

Introduction

"Knock, knock!"
"Who's there?"
"Shirley..."
"Shirley who?"
"Shirley you know who I am by now!"

There's nothing like a knock, knock joke for capturing six- and seven-year-olds' sense of fun. The joke lies in the incongruity which makes the familiar seem unfamiliar. In this particular joke the person on the other side of the door doesn't know a "Shirley", but it's not Shirley at all...it's someone who has been known for ages but with quite a different name.

At this age, the world seems to be full of new possibilities, and children are at a sort of threshold. They are becoming more established at school and many new skills are beginning to come together. Children are able to manage greater independence in many areas of their lives but they still need plenty of support from home in dealing with the ordinary stresses of life. Perhaps the greatest challenge for them now is to find ways to put aside babyish ways in order to explore the exciting challenges that middle childhood has to offer.

More formal work at school is supplemented and fed by a child's natural spirit of enquiry and by imagination. The ordinary experiences of daily life are full of richness and meaning, and are being shaped according to the child's emerging personality. It can be a challenge for parents to stay in touch and appropriately in control while allowing sufficient leeway for new relationships to develop in their child's life. If parents allow themselves to get to know their child afresh by pausing to look again, as if from a slight emotional distance, at their child's development, it is possible to imagine what the world is like from a child's point of view. All parents have been children themselves, and so their own memories of being six and seven can be a very valuable resource for understanding. On the other hand, children are inevitably different from their parents. Their personalities are not only unique to themselves but also influenced by the technologies and media of the twenty-first century which bring the world right into their living rooms in ways which seemed unimaginable a generation ago.

As children develop and grow up there can be mixed feelings for parents and children alike about the emotional adjustments that need to be made. This is a major theme explored in this book. From a parent's point of view there is an enormous sense of satisfaction to be gained in helping children to develop new skills and abilities such as reading and number work. Children are beginning to think in more sophisticated ways and orient themselves better in relation to time and space. Physical skills and coordination are growing apace and they can do more in the way of looking after themselves, taking greater responsibility for such tasks as washing and dressing. New relationships and friendships are forming and taking on great importance, and this can help parents to feel freer to pursue interests of their own. Parents usually feel proud when their children are thriving in these ways, but they may feel sadness, also, at needing to say goodbye to the intimacy of the earlier, more dependent years. From a child's point of view, there is a need, now, to put aside some of the more passionate feelings associated with family relationships. Children are faced with the challenge of packing away their earlier experience, rather like a metaphorical packed lunch, to provide inner sustenance to keep them going as they face the challenges of learning in school, making friendships and coping with the wider world.

Taking stock of the incredible pace of a child's development, it can be hard to believe that this is the same child as the one who so recently just started school. "Six going on sixteen!" is how one mother described her daughter, adding that already she could imagine her as an adult-to-be, a miniature adolescent. So it can be helpful to remind oneself that in fact a six-year-old is still only a third of the way through the long human journey towards adulthood. Another of the themes explored in this book is the tension created for the child when he or she no longer feels small but is not yet very big: "smalley-big", as one six-year-old so succinctly put it. It is sometimes quite salutary to remember that a six-year-old's apparent competence is, at times, only paper thin and can be easily punctured by the ordinary stresses and strains of life.

Between their sixth and eighth birthdays children gradually give up more magical kinds of thinking in favour of more rational, logical ways of seeing the world. They begin to realize that success cannot be gained by charm alone; on the contrary, hard work is expected, and this can be enjoyed, but can bring with it stress and a fear of failure. Children's attraction to reality and achievement is tempered by imagination and an increased ability to symbolize and represent experience through language, play and pretending. When teachers are in tune with children of this age they can really mobilize their more mature side to collaborate with their more childish selves through creative class projects. Many primary trained teachers find the six- to seven-year-old age group particularly rewarding to teach because their imaginative selves are so accessible alongside their enthusiasm to learn skills and facts.

The key aim of this book is to bring to life some of the many facets of the experience of being six or seven. Some typical dilemmas of this age group are explored along with some thoughts about related issues for parents. There will, of course, be areas of overlap with children who are five or even eight or so, as every child is an individual and matures at his or her own pace. Essentially we are thinking here about the phase of development at the beginning of middle childhood which is sometimes referred to as the "latency" period. If children are reasonably well supported in their home lives this tends to be a period of steady growth, learning and consolidation.

For the sake of clarity, a teacher or parent is sometimes referred to as "she" but what is said is meant to apply to fathers, carers and teachers of both genders as well as mothers.

1

A Changing Sense of Self

Making sense of who you are is very much work in progress when you are six or seven. Physical and emotional changes go hand in hand, and although the external changes are very clear to see, internal changes are less apparent. In this chapter we will take a look at the ways in which six- and seven-year-olds are developing new ways of relating to the world. As their perspectives change, so too do their capacities to learn, to understand and to represent their experience.

Children are doing a great deal of growing between their sixth and eighth birthdays. Their rounder, cuddly little child appearance gradually gives way to something more robust. Top front milk teeth tend to have fallen out, but the new second teeth which will last a lifetime are not quite fully formed, giving an impression of gaps yet to be filled. So it is at an emotional level. Infancy, as represented by the milk teeth, has been left behind but adulthood is still a long way off. In between, there is a lot of learning to do. Children are developing in coordination and balance, acquiring fine motor skills like writing and drawing, amassing knowledge and information at an astonishing pace and gaining experience of all sorts, both social and intellectual. All of this is likely to be, at times, at the cost of some stress and strain which calls for sensitive adult support. Children are likely to compare themselves with others no matter how much we may wish to persuade them not to. Competition and rivalry are part of the human condition and children of this age often strive to fit in to be like the others. Some will want to be the best at something. This brings with it worries about not being able to manage, or an unwillingness to risk failure. Rather than the overconfident "I can do it" attitude more characteristic of toddlers, this age group is coming to terms with the need for determination and effort to make headway in life. A great deal of sympathetic encouragement is often needed to help children persevere in the face of difficulty.

It's good to talk

A capacity to discuss things and to express thoughts and ideas in conversation is a fantastic asset. Spoken language is a vehicle for getting to know other people and becoming known by others. If children have had experiences, over time, of being listened to, thought about and understood, they will now be asking all sorts of interesting questions and articulating novel ideas. Children's statements can often convey something well beyond the literal words once they start to enjoy language.

Henry was a shy and serious six-year-old who had been finding it hard to settle down again to the routine of school after the long summer holidays. He was just beginning to get used to his new status as a "top infant", along with a new classroom and a new teacher. After school he was very tired and spoke very little, but during tea he volunteered some new knowledge about the school building. "D'you know," he told his parents, "when I was in reception class I didn't even know where the Resources Room was... I didn't even know there was an upstairs!" Henry's sense that he was entering a larger world came through this simple statement, and his parents felt he was telling them something about discovering new resources in himself as well as at school.

On other occasions Henry's typically six-year-old tendency to ask pressing questions kept his parents on their toes. "I just don't get it! Where *do* people come from?" was one such question. His parents wondered whether this was an enquiry about a matter of geography, biology, or human relationships. When he asked, on another occasion, "How exactly do aeroplanes stay up?" his father tried to respond with a detailed explanation, only to find that Henry's attention quickly wandered off elsewhere. Perhaps for Henry the point was to share his sense of wonder about the world rather than to uncover scientific fact.

Six- and seven-year-olds are discovering that language can be used to convey complicated ideas. Language can now be used in a metaphorical as well as a literal way, paving the way for sharing jokes and imaginative games as part of making friends. Of course, language can also be used under the sway of less friendly feelings, to manipulate or hurt. Swear words are often discovered and highly prized by children of this age as something dangerous, exciting and definitely prohibited. They know they are not supposed to use them, but they like to provoke and test out adult responses.

Changing perspectives

At around the age of seven there are some very significant developmental changes to the ways children are able to think. Abstract thinking becomes more possible, with most children understanding, for example, that not only does "3" represent three things, but also there can be an idea of "threeness" which can be manipulated in the mind together with other numbers to perform additions and subtractions. We adults, who call this process "mental arithmetic", rarely stop to think what a sophisticated operation this is.

Children of this age are starting to grasp the idea of place value. Now a child has to bear in mind that 3 can actually mean 30 or 300, depending on whether it is in the "units", "tens" or "hundreds" column. It is often easier to grasp abstract ideas when they relate to something better known. When Sabah was doing some number work with her mother, she told her, "Units are like – not many, like when you stay at home." For Sabah, "units" were linked to thoughts about being one of only two children at home, whereas "tens" and "hundreds" reminded her of being at school. Sabah's way of thinking shows that children make sense of abstract concepts by making a link with what is on their mind already. Often, what is on their mind is their family. When children feel thought about and listened to by those they love and care for most, they learn more readily. Worries or concerns which are home-related can inhibit learning.

Children's understanding of the world is informed by a great deal of practice with measuring of various kinds, which helps them to begin to orient themselves in space and time. Measuring height and length is straightforward enough, but it is only at around age seven that children can really begin to understand concepts such as volume and capacity, which require two factors to be taken into account at the same time. In other words, three-dimensional thinking is required. Children are now more likely to understand that liquids do not change in volume when they are poured from one container to another of a different shape. Similarly, if shown two balls of plasticine of the same size, they can understand that rolling one into a sausage shape does not alter the overall amount of plasticine. A younger child will probably focus on one dimension such as the height of the liquid in the container, or the length of the sausage-shaped piece of plasticine, but the slightly older child will see that if nothing is added or taken away, the volume remains the same. This development in thinking comes in due course if children feel secure enough to experiment and to make these sorts of discoveries through play. At an emotional level this security is linked to a sense of being remembered and thought about in a flexible way in the minds of the adults who care for them as they move around fitting in with different social environments of home, friendships and the classroom. They come to experience themselves as having a more consistent identity which moves with them between situations in which different things are expected of them.

Social understanding, or empathy, plays a very important part in six- and seven-year-olds' ability to think and learn. When children can put themselves, imaginatively, into the shoes of others in order to get to know them, they are broadening their horizons in a very meaningful way. Empathy is an essential aspect of making and keeping friendships because it is part of getting to know about others' lives and cultures and, by implication, what it feels like to be human. But most six- and seven-year-olds can be empathetic, flexible thinkers for only a few moments in an average day. Especially if they are tired, they are more likely to be irritable and inflexible when asked to see things from any perspective other than their own. This theme is explored in an amusing little book by David McKee entitled *Two Monsters*. These monsters live on opposite sides of a mountain, which serves as an obstacle to them seeing eye-to-eye in more ways than one. They cannot agree about anything until their squabbling leads to knocking the mountain down. Finally they come to see that their views had more in common than they had supposed.

Children of this age are, indeed, beginning to understand differing points of view. In a test devised to explore this aspect of development (and also, by coincidence, involving a mountain), a psychologist showed seven-year-old William a three-dimensional model of a mountainous landscape. A doll was placed on the opposite side of the model, facing William, and he was asked to describe what the doll could see. William found this a difficult task and he decided the best thing to do was to turn the model round so that the doll's view was roughly the same as his own. William's approach to the task was typical of how children begin to understand new situations. We all come to know the new with reference to the more familiar, and in this way our expectations when faced with a new situation are coloured by earlier experiences. It is, therefore, understandable that children's ways of relating to their teacher will be based on their pool of experience of relationships with the adults they know best, their parents, while relating to classmates will initially be based on the way in which earlier relationships such as those with siblings have been negotiated in the family.

A sense of balance

Physical and emotional balance are required in order to learn to ride a proper bicycle, and the processes involved illustrate the sorts of dilemmas involved in greater independence. Learning to ride a two-wheeler bike can be an important rite of passage, and children who have mastered this skill can take their place alongside the older children without shame. On the other hand, as the pace of propulsion away from the parental orbit accelerates, parents are often left feeling somewhat like the discarded stabilizers. In order to learn to ride properly, children have to learn a number of new skills. They have to learn how a bicycle works and how to use their body and mind in a coordinated way. At an emotional level they have to tolerate setbacks and difficulties, and, above all, be able to accept help from an adult. Most importantly, a child needs to let go of the idea that new skills can be acquired magically by simply wishing them so. This can lead to turbulent feelings in the learner.

Gemma had been watching her eight-year-old brother riding his bike with his friends and was convinced that it would be easy. Her mother had taken her to the park for a lesson without stabilizers, but Gemma did not want her mother to hold on to the back of the bike to help her as she got up speed. Understandably, Gemma found it difficult to coordinate pedalling, steering and balancing at first. She was very wobbly and fell several times, but she seemed to feel that the difficulty in getting her balance was her mother's fault for not helping in the right way. What her mother knew was that she was holding on to the back of the bike to help her daughter, but Gemma was convinced that she was actually holding her back. Gemma's fury with her mother seemed to be fuelled by the pain of her sore knees and elbows. She would not let herself be comforted, choosing instead to push the hurt feelings into her mother, who could see that Gemma was suffering but had to tolerate being seen as unhelpful.

It took a great deal of negotiation, perseverance and several trips to the park before Gemma could really manage by herself. Like many children she needed a week or two to cool off from the humiliating experience of not being able to learn instantly. Once she had mastered the art of riding, Gemma's manner became much more confident. She loved the sense of freedom and the exhilaration of speed which bike riding brought. Gemma's anger with her mother soon subsided and led to a subtly changed relationship, based on getting alongside her. Family cycling trips became an enjoyable weekend activity that included all four family members. Conflict was not entirely out of the picture, however, with Gemma being very determined to be the one in the lead and, particularly, to win all the races against her older brother.

Right and wrong

In the main, children know, by now, when they are pretending and when they are not, and along with this comes a better developed sense of reality. They are more able to say what the truth is and how it is different from a lie. Whereas one five-year-old asserted that a lie was a "naughty story", his older brother knew that a lie was "not telling the truth". This is an important distinction, which shows that the more mature child sees lying as a sort of choice. Implicit, also, is the idea that it is possible to find out the truth by looking at the evidence, including the evidence of feelings.

It is important that children come to make a clear distinction between right and wrong at this age. They are usually working out aspects of this theme in the games they play with others, by themselves with their toy figures, and in the stories and films they like. Having some clarity on questions of morality is the basis of social cooperation and children of this age tend to want to fit in and to be accepted. But this process is complicated by the mixed feelings of love and hate which are common to all of us. Everyone has angry, hurtful and unkind impulses at times; it simply cannot be helped. As adults, we are generally aware that such feelings do not, in themselves, cause actual harm to others. Children, on the other hand, can tend to blame themselves when things go wrong. The logic may go something like this: I had a nasty feeling so I am bad and I made a bad thing happen. If, for example, parents separate, or a sister or brother becomes ill, a six- or seven-year-old may wonder whose fault it is, and may be inclined to blame him- or herself.

Sorting out reality and fantasy

Children's sense of identity is still rather fluid at this age, as they move with ease between the worlds of rational understanding and imagination. There are wide variations between children, with some beginning to be keen on facts, figures, rules and information, whereas others are temperamentally more inclined towards creativity, ideas and pretending. In the main these two different strands are discernible in the same six-year-old at different times. Henry, for example, so full of wonder at one moment, could be a very concrete thinker the next. Examining the label on a new packet of vests one morning, he commented with derision, "What's this? Two sleeveless vests! Well, how are you supposed to get those on?!" Taking things a little too literally, Henry had convinced himself that his mother had bought him vests without armholes. This misunderstanding could also have stemmed from Henry's wish to be like his father, who was inclined to be a bit of a social critic.

Taking things too literally is all very well, but parents may feel concerned if their child is too caught up in a world of his or her own. *I Am Really a Princess* is the title of a delightful storybook for six-year-olds by Carol Diggory Shields. This story is about a little girl's insistence that reality is as she would wish it to be. She insists that she ought not to be asked to tidy up nor be expected to make allowances for her baby brother's needs. In the story, the heroine's kindly parents indulge her fantasies up to a point. They are willing to suspend disbelief, as many parents do. But by the time children are six or seven more reality-based behaviour is generally expected. On the other hand a certain amount of creative make-believe lends considerable charm to children's personalities, making them a lot of fun to be with, and parents are often happy to go along with the magic of childhood imagination. A small child's life is not complete without fantasy and fairy stories as these are ways of expressing hopes, wishes, fears and disappointments.

Myths such as those of Father Christmas and the tooth fairy are very appealing to both children and adults alike. This may be because they support the fantasy of ideal parents who are endlessly giving and generous, asking nothing in return. In reality, of course, parents have to impose restrictions, rules and limits in a child's best interests, but what a pity this is so, we might feel. By this age, children generally have a pretty good idea that the tooth fairy does not really exist but they may still go along with the idea as long as parents do, simply because it is fun.

When Sabah was six years old she told her sister, in confidence, that she had worked out what the tooth fairy does with the teeth she takes. If it is a yellow tooth it is simply thrown away, she explained, and the owner does not get any money for it, but if it is a good, clean tooth the fairy uses it to build herself a castle and pays one pound for it. It seemed to Sabah that when she found her one pound under the pillow (ostensibly from the tooth fairy), it was evidence that her efforts to be a good girl who looks after her teeth were being recognized and rewarded. The tooth perhaps stood for an idea about a no-longer-needed part of her which, however, could be used as a resource or building block for further developments. One year on, Sabah, now aged seven and a half, was becoming much more of a realist, and she insisted that her parents tell her the truth. Furthermore, she let them know that her friends said the rate had now increased to two pounds for a well kept molar!

2

A Place in the Family

Home is still at the heart of any child's identity at six or seven. Life at home provides children with a sense of belonging, continuity and acceptance which makes it possible to begin to face the challenges of the outside world. In our complex and changing society the range of what might be considered "ordinary" families is enormous. Whereas the majority of children still live with a mother, father and a sibling or two, it is not at all unusual for children to have parents who live in different households. Many children grow up in single-parent families, stepfamilies or extended kinship arrangements. Parental partnerships may be formed between couples of the same gender, or arrangements for raising children may include a very active role for grandparents. Each sort of family brings with it its own strengths and difficulties, but it needs to be acknowledged that a family may take on many forms.

Many Western schools are proudly multicultural; families have migrated from around the world during this or previous generations, bringing to their new country a rich diversity of cultures. Faith communities and ethnic groupings may contribute to a family's way of defining themselves. In this way particular circumstances contribute to the sense of home which individual six- and seven-year-olds carry within themselves. On the other hand, now that children are established at school, home values are no longer the sole organizing factors in their lives. There is an old Arabic saying that "Men resemble their times more than their fathers," and this has relevance for the six- and seven-year-olds of today. They may be beginning to see that although they start from very different places, they are also part of a community of six- and seven-year-olds with common interests. Whatever the family setting in which children live, they will be alert to the ways in which those who care for them relate to one another, and children will be studying what makes them "tick".

Goodbye to being the baby

"Smalley-big" children are beginning to give up some of the intimate close-ness with parents which they enjoyed when they were younger, in favour of friendships and activities in the outside world. There is still a wide variation between children in their ability to separate from their parents. Some will appear completely undaunted by the idea of greater independence, but on the whole it is more realistic to expect children to oscillate between being confident at one moment and less so the next. This is because the gains of independence are possible only alongside an ability to manage loss. Children will have had some practice in managing loss in the context of earlier relation-ships. Giving up being the tiny baby-at-the-breast in order to move on to try out solid foods, and the process of weaning, has been a sort of prototype for later experiences of renunciation. Later, there has been the move to nursery, kindergarten or playgroup, which has meant giving up being exclusively a home child, while more recently, the child has been settling in to big school and adapting to being one of a large group of children. All of these changes and others – perhaps, say, of moving to a new neighbourhood – will have been unsettling and taken time to absorb.

Experiences of transition involve the joy and excitement of the new, tempered by poignancy and sadness at the loss of what has had to be given up. There is often the reality that a child has to give up being the baby, to make way for another baby, and this can lead to complex feelings including jealousy, rivalry and competitiveness. The most obvious targets for such feelings are younger brothers and sisters, who may be felt to have stolen Mummy away. Even when there has been no actual new baby, the feeling for children of parents who are simply taken up with other matters may be a feeling that someone else has taken what was formerly theirs.

Nadine was an only child who was used to having her parents' attention to herself, so it was rather a shock to her when her family went on holiday with some friends who had a four-month-old baby. She found the shared domestic arrangements rather a strain, particularly around mealtimes. In her own home, Nadine was used to being a focus for attention when she sat down for dinner with her father, mother and teenage stepsister. So it was upsetting for her to have to share her parents' attention with this other family. It was bad enough that her father kept talking with the other father about lots of adult matters that she did not understand, but worse still, her mother would not let her help herself to yoghurts from the fridge because the provisions were for both families. It seemed to Nadine that, by contrast, baby Aliya in the other family had things all her own way. She was constantly in the arms of one parent or another and constantly (or so it seemed) being fed and made a fuss of. It was enough to put any six-year-old in a bad mood.

Nadine would not eat her dinner and repeatedly interrupted the adults' conversation with requests for yoghurt. She rocked on her chair and banged her knife and fork on her plate in an irritating manner. Eventually her mother, who had been gently urging her to eat her dinner, commented: "Nadine, for someone who is six you really are being a bit of a baby." Nadine was incensed. "I'm NOT a baby!" she shouted in angry indignation and she continued thus as she was taken out of the room to calm down. Outside in the corridor Nadine continued with what by now had all the hallmarks of a toddler's tantrum: "But I'm NOT a baby, I'm not!" Slowly, the tone of Nadine's complaint altered, until her mother could discern that it had become a bitter lament. "But I'm NOT a baby," and the tears began to roll down her face as her mother at last understood. Only now was she able to give and for Nadine to accept a cuddle, which acknowledged just how painful it can be to grow up and leave infancy behind.

In this example, Nadine was faced with a dilemma typical of her new status as a six-year-old. She was not yet an adult, being unable to participate in the adult conversations, nor was she able to help herself to food from the fridge, as this was another privilege reserved for adults. Yet she was also aware that the role of baby was not available to her either. She was expected to be something else, a "mature" six-year-old, and while this was something she could generally manage, on this occasion she had been overwhelmed by feelings that there was no place for her to be. Her mother's cuddle communicated more than words might do on this occasion, and recognized that Nadine was still a *bit* of a baby, but that was OK. It is very helpful to keep in mind children's dependent side alongside their competent self.

As Nadine's mother found, there are mixed feelings for the parents to manage too. There is great pride in having a more articulate and independent child, but development is rarely straightforward. It is hard to strike a balance between recognizing that as a parent you are still very much needed, and being willing to let go so that your child can explore the possibility of having a little more life of his or her own.

Competition and rivalry

It is universal for children to mind when they have to share the attention of their parents with others, and at this age this is likely to be played out between brothers and sisters. Competitive and rivalrous feelings are a healthy asset in fair measure. This is part of what makes for determination to succeed and perseverance in the face of setbacks, as in the example of Gemma, who was learning to ride a bike. If her brother could do it, she thought, then she would do it too, but even better if possible.

Six- or seven-year-old children who are the older child in a family are likely to make the most of their position at times to boost their sense of superiority, but if this tips too much into a habit of riding roughshod over the feelings of a younger sibling, parents usually feel this is unhelpful. In fact it is often the case that children who are excessively scornful of babies or younger children are likely to fear that their own lack of experience or incomplete understanding will be greeted with contempt by others. So when children consistently humiliate a younger child it may well be an attempt to rid themselves of their own feelings of insecurity. They probably feel, at some level, that their own dependence is contemptible. Parents can help children see that it takes a long time to learn things, and there is no shame in having to struggle along the way. Scornful children often fear to expose their own need for help because they do not expect to be met with kindness or understanding. For this reason, although parents will be drawn towards supporting the younger, more vulnerable child, it is worth bearing in mind that a contemptuous older child needs support and understanding too. Trying to help a hurtful child to think about the other's point of view will be far more helpful than punishment in the long run.

Sibling relationships are often stormy but learning to negotiate and manage strong feelings offers a source of great enrichment. Sharing stories can be a good way of exploring these themes. *Get Lost, Laura!* by Jennifer Northway examines an older sister's wish to get away from an annoying younger sister. When Laura really does get lost, the older sister tries to make amends. Sibling relationships of a less than pleasant kind are also explored in the Horrid Henry series of books by Francesca Simon. These books are popular with independent readers of around seven years who like to explore some nasty impulses of their own at a safe distance and laugh at Henry's antics.

In real life jealousy and rivalry between siblings can sometimes feel very raw and this can be deeply upsetting to parents, who often wish there was some way to keep the peace. Working out how to intervene in disputes between siblings where there are two or more conflicting accounts of events can be very exhausting. Children of this age often have an exaggerated sense of fair play but a fixed view of things when they are angry. In spite of this, perseverance and consistency in the adults will probably move things on in due course. It is worth remembering that families offer a sort of laboratory for working out relationships and strong feelings. The hard work put in at home carries over into the school setting and helps with the all-important task of making and keeping friends.

Identifying with parents

Now that the more obviously dependent relationships of infancy are fading, and there are such huge advances in children's abilities to use and to understand spoken language, many other changes are noticeable. Six- and seven-year-olds are looking for opportunities to get alongside their parents in a more friendly way, and there is often a gender divide, with girls taking a greater interest in the things that Mum does, and enjoying a new kind of companionship with her. Long chats and shopping trips, for example, can make daughters feel pretty grown-up. Boys of this age begin to show a marked preference for doing things with Dad and are becoming interested in what it means to have a male identity. Having private time with Dad is particularly prized as a chance to study his admired qualities. Mums may have to tolerate being second best for a while. If dads are sports enthusiasts, this will be the age when their sons are likely to be joining clubs to learn the basic skills. Football clubs are very popular with boys, even more so when Dad shows an interest in supporting on the sidelines. Girls, on the other hand, may be drawn towards dancing, drama or whatever else their parents and friends go in for. Taking part in activities which have their parents' support seems to appeal universally. Children benefit enormously when parents take an interest in them, but it is important for parents to keep a sense of proportion, not to push their child too far, and to allow for the great diversity of children's personalities. There are always some sports-mad girls and more domestically oriented boys among any group. Children's interests can wax and wane at this age, and if children feel too pressurized it may put them off. This is even more likely if the activities take place at the weekend when children sometimes prefer to relax away from formal demands.

Past, present and future

Family groupings have one important thing in common. They consist of people of different generations. Children around this age are interested in the passage of time and the alterations that time brings. In a lovely, beautifully illustrated storybook for children entitled *Once There Were Giants* by Martin Waddell and Penny Dale, the authors explore children's interest in the fact that their parents were children once and that they, themselves, will eventually be adults. Children of this age are beginning to be able to learn to tell the time on a clock face and developing quite a fascination with the meanings of time.

Rochelle had been studying "famous people" for a project at school and she spoke a lot to her parents about Mary Seacole and how she had rescued soldiers in the Crimean war. Her train of thought about "long ago" prompted her to ask her mum why she listened to old-fashioned music. Mum replied that it reminded her of when she was younger. After a pause for thought, Rochelle asked whether that meant that *she* would get to like that sort of music when she was older. On further reflection, however, she decided, "No. I will still like Jennifer Lopez and Beyoncé because they will be old-fashioned by then."

Children are developing a sense of family history, and in getting to know their grandparents come to understand more about getting older and having a lifespan. Inevitably they will have some questions about death and begin to see that this is something irreversible. Some children go through a phase of being very shaken by this discovery, feeling that nothing can be as solid and certain as it was before.

Lauren was a sensitive seven-year-old who was understandably upset when the family's elderly cat died. Her sadness was mixed with anger: "If I could find out who invented the word 'dead'," she told her mother, "I would just kill them." Poor Lauren wished there was a way to get rid of an awareness of death, but she was helped by her family to see the value of ritual and mourning. Her parents decided that they would bury this much loved family pet in the back garden, with a respectful little ceremony which included her brothers and a visiting aunt. It was Lauren's idea that they all sing a song. She could not think of one about a cat so she made one up. There was something valuable in coming together with loved ones, which made it possible for Lauren to face her loss. Within a week, Lauren's thoughts were already turning towards a wish for a new kitten.

We can see that both Lauren and Rochelle had been doing some deep thinking about time, putting together different strands of their experience in ways which are characteristic of children of this age.

Parents are only human

When she was younger, Lauren had felt secure in the belief that parents could put right just about any difficulty. If she grazed her knee, Mum would put "magic" cream on the wound and make it better, or if she was frightened a cuddle would generally be enough to save the day. Now, things were a little different. She knew more about the complexity of the world and recognized, sadly, that her parents could not prevent her cat from dying. In the same way, they could not learn her spellings for her, or stop her best friend being unkind and hurting her feelings. Lauren was in fact feeling rather disillusioned, realizing that parents can offer love, guidance and support but they are not all-powerful as she had once supposed.

This theme is explored in a series of sensitively observed stories for young readers, including *But You Promised!* by Bel Mooney. The heroine, Kitty, wants her parents' guarantee on matters which cannot really be settled simply. In one of the stories, Kitty does not want to go to the doctor's for an injection and makes her parents promise that it will not hurt too much. When the injection does hurt, Kitty is cross with her father for letting her down. In the story, Dad talks to Kitty kindly:

> "One thing you have to learn," Dad tells Kitty with a warm smile, "Parents don't control everything. When grown-ups say 'I promise' they usually mean 'I hope'."

Like Kitty, children are discovering that just as parents do not know everything, they also make mistakes. It is unwise for parents to make promises which cannot be kept. Parents do not always respond to their children as, ideally, they would like to. For example, they may find themselves responding to their child in a bad-tempered way, or they may falsely accuse the child of some misdemeanour. No parent is perfect. But all is not lost if they can share with their child that on reflection they are sorry. In fact there can be some value in this, as children begin to learn the value of self-reflection when their parents set an example.

While parents are not all-powerful, they do need to remain in control and there are inevitably times when their authority is sorely tested. It would be surprising if a child of six or seven was not stubborn, irritable, contrary and belligerent from time to time. When this happens parents need to be able to stand their ground, to say "No" and to mean it. They also need to bear the resulting fallout. Parents sometimes find it difficult to put up with the unpopularity which can come from setting limits. If parents experienced over-harsh discipline when they were younger, they can come to feel that they are doing damage by being firm with their own children. Nonetheless, setting fair limits is fundamentally an expression of love and concern.

There are bound to be times when family life is difficult. If there are strains in the relationship between the parents, this is bound to take its toll on the children in the family. There may be external stress such as work problems, financial difficulties, illness or a bereavement. However, children are generally quite resilient, and if parents can be sufficiently supported by partners, family, friends and community to work through and eventually get over the difficulties, the children usually bounce back too. A certain amount of adversity is part of life, but if problems persist and become entrenched it may be wise to seek help. Your family doctor or your child's school will often be the best first port of call, and can help with referral to more specialized services if these are needed.

3

The Experience of School

Ready for school

By the age of six it is fairly universal for children to wish to transform their passionate, volatile behaviour into orderliness and achievement. This is by and large gratifying for all concerned. School, with its emphasis on consistency and predictable routines, is welcomed as a place where growing competencies can be demonstrated. Parental support is still very much needed, but children may not show their need of this as obviously as in the past. On the contrary, the kind of non-verbal message children may give their parents at the start of the school day might be expressed as "I love you, but now go away." Such self-assurance is evidence that a degree of stability has been achieved, but how has it come about?

Children's engagement with the world is based upon their earlier experiences with a primary carer, usually the mother. Slowly a child's world expands to include the father, siblings and other members of the immediate family. The toddler's emerging sense of self has its base in repeated experiences of being sensitively responded to and understood. In other words, development takes place in the context of relationships. If all goes reasonably well, toddlers become increasingly interested in those around them and the relationships between them. Three- or four-year-old children may be able to play alongside other children, but this will be in a rather egocentric way with limited scope for negotiation. The move to school at the age of four or five means that children need to muster all their resources to cope with managing the demands of the school day as one of a class of 30 or so. They will need to learn a certain amount of sensitivity to others, and it is to be hoped that this has been practised within the family, at playgroup or nursery, in adult-mediated encounters with other children. Natural competitiveness fuels a drive to succeed, while a capacity to learn from parents will have prepared children for the need to pay attention to their teacher. In spite of all this preparation, and even in the face of apparent confidence, every parent knows that a six-year-old is still vulnerable and dependent.

As Ryan and his mother arrived at five minutes to nine on one windy Monday morning, the playground was thronging with parents, children and pushchairs. Six or seven children in Ryan's class had already lined up, jostling for position as they waited for Mrs Campbell, their teacher, to arrive. Ryan's friend, James, had brought his football, and the friends chatted about who would play in which position at playtime. Another boy, Jason, appeared from the crowd, approaching Ryan a little too closely, pulling his hood and prodding his face in a rough greeting. Unlike the other children, Jason was not accompanied by an adult, and did not pay much attention to Ryan's mother when she asked him not to poke other children in the face. Just then, the teacher arrived and the mass of children suddenly transformed themselves into an orderly line, which snaked off, good humouredly, into the school building.

As she kissed her son goodbye, Ryan's mother, like many parents, had to bear the fact that her son had to find his own way and to manage being a member of this large class of children. She could remember her own infant school days and how she had suffered at times with a sense of being an outsider. On reflection she wondered whether some of this had led to her intervening with Jason and being a bit over-protective rather than letting Ryan sort things out for himself. After all, part of what growing up is about is learning to manage temporary adversity by holding on to the memory of good experiences. Parents may not always think about it this way, but when they hand their child over to school they transfer considerable responsibility for their child's well-being to a relatively unknown adult, the teacher, which is not an easy thing to do.

Relationship to the teacher

A child's class teacher becomes a very important person to him or her and a central authority figure outside of the family. More than this, she is an emotional anchor during the school day. Children draw on their earlier relationships as a resource for understanding new ones, and the relationship with the teacher will inevitably be coloured by experiences of parents, grandparents and other important adults. Even though children of this age are less likely to expect their teacher to respond to them as their mother does, they will need and want to be noticed as an individual and to feel valued as such. The quality of the teacher's attention will be the key organizing factor in their experience of learning at school. If the teacher has a warm personality a child is likely to develop a special bond with her, regarding her with awe and admiration. An admired teacher is often the subject of intense scrutiny from pupils, who will be fascinated by her ways of doing things. The stronger is a child's wish to please her and to succeed, the more likely the child is to fear failure, and this may lead to seeing the teacher as quite severe or frightening at times. There is a subtle shift of gear at age six and children are aware that going to school is no longer an achievement in itself. Children are now expected to get on in a more focused and purposeful way. Results are expected and these are achieved only by application and hard work.

It is important to children that their teacher is someone who can keep order and maintain a steady, respectful atmosphere in the classroom. In this matter her ways of relating will be more geared towards the needs of the group and less towards the individual's own needs than any particular child might wish. The match between child and teacher is a complex one and may contain many elements, positive and negative. When parents weigh these up in their minds, an essential question they will tend to ask themselves is "Does this teacher create a sense of security in the classroom which enables my child to learn?"

It can help to overcome the natural sadness felt at losing a "home child" if the child is happy and feels safe with the teacher. But it is fairly universal for parents to worry about their child's move from a familiar teacher to a new one for the following school year. Will this new teacher be too strict or too soft? Will she deal with any potential disruptive goings on in the classroom while being accessible and fair-minded? It can sometimes happen that there is a mismatch between teacher and child, and if it does, the headteacher is usually best placed to arbitrate. Sorting things out generally depends on a mutual willingness for parent, teacher and child to get to know each other. It may take a little time, but a feeling of supportive partnership between home and school is bound to be in a child's best interests.

Many children of this age become absorbed in studying their teachers, often taking in every detail of their attitudes and mannerisms. Louis often went through a ritual of "taking the register" before going to sleep, just like his teacher did. Sensing that this was important to Louis, his mother indulged him. At his request she regularly found herself answering an imaginary register in 30 different voices before Louis would go to sleep. School habits and ways of doing things can become very important to six- and seven-year-olds, with strategies that work well at school being tried at home. For example, Stephen's mother noticed that he would try sitting up straight and putting his hand up when trying to get attention from his parents, whereas Melissa, who had sometimes called her teacher "Mummy" in reception class, was now inclined to make the mistake of calling her mother by her teacher's name. This sort of mistake shows us just how very important school ways have become. It also underlines what a lot of effort children put in to the matter of getting adult attention. In school this may be hard won and require very particular strategies.

Difficulties can arise when there are frequent changes of teacher. Sonia became distressed and reluctant to go to school when her teacher's illness led to her having a series of supply teachers. Her mother felt almost cruel to force her child to go to school when she felt that Sonia's experiences were not of a good quality at that time. She went to discuss this with the headteacher, who was able to arrange for Sonia to have more small group work with a familiar classroom assistant to help her through this unsettling period. Sonia's difficulties soon subsided once her regular teacher returned to school safe and well.

Being one child in a big class

It is really very hard for children in a large class to wait their turn, to put their hands up again and again and not be chosen to answer. Many children add emphasis with groans and straining noises in sheer enthusiasm to answer a question. It can be very demoralizing if, after a long and eager wait to be chosen, their answer turns out not to be what was wanted. Most children want to be noticed by the teacher and when there is a good chance of this happening, it will be a spur to achievement. Vying for the teacher's attention is sometimes a carry-over from home, where children compete with siblings for a special place with mother or father. Managing a long school day as one of so many children can be difficult to get used to and children of this age will need a store of inner resources to help them get through.

Rules, procedures and routines in the classroom are very reassuring and help children to develop a feeling of knowing what to expect. Familiarity with school routines is enormously encouraging for children in a large class where fears of potential chaos are often lurking not far beneath the surface.

Nor do such fears exist solely in the minds of the children. Skilled teachers harness children's satisfaction with rules which promote cooperation and a sense of order. For example, in Mrs Campbell's class there was a system of table points awarded to groups of children who kept their communal equipment (pencils, scissors and suchlike) in exemplary order. Points could earn a reward known as "Golden time". This was a time, at the end of the school week, when they could play a game or other activity of their choice. Similarly, Mrs Campbell kept a jar by the classroom door into which "class marbles" were accumulated when the children lined up nicely or achieved some other goal as a whole group. The children knew that they had to earn a certain number of marbles per week to get "Golden time" on Fridays. These simple, behavioural strategies mobilized the children's naturally competitive instincts in a productive way. They began to develop a feel for group endeavour.

Children of this age love to accumulate evidence of themselves as "good" and law-abiding, but it sometimes suits them to have a naughty child in their class. Their own wishes to misbehave can then be disowned and located in this other child. Telling tales in order to ingratiate themselves with the teacher is something which can happen quite subtly and have a damaging effect on group cohesion. Good teachers do their best to defuse the sorts of dynamic in which particular children are seen in fixed ways. For example, they will play to the strengths of pupils with special educational needs and encourage shy children to express themselves with more assertiveness. The ebb and flow of classroom relationships offers many opportunities for children to explore different sides to their personalities, as they watch and learn about how members of the class group are treated.

Lesson time

Effective learning for children of this age makes links between their experiences of life at home and at school. Education of the whole child also takes account of links between their awareness of reality and their imaginative lives. In fact at six or seven, children's natural tendency to play and pretend can offer opportunities for some wonderful, creative project work. Work can be fun, and fun can be work, and if the fun is extended to involve parents as well, schools are on to a winning formula for promoting learning.

Through the Dragon's Eye is a popular BBC *Look and Read* programme in the UK, shown in ten weekly episodes, which spawns a whole range of imaginative learning opportunities in the classroom. Mrs Campbell adapted the story to make an imaginative link between the children's homes and school. Once the register had been completed, lesson time began with a routine which was both educational and fun.

"Now," announced Mrs Campbell, "Let's see who took Gorwen home last night!" There was a visible frisson of excitement. The children loved this routine. Many seemed to wake up for the first time that morning. Gorwen was a large, red, plush toy dragon belonging to Mrs Campbell, whose name came from the character of the same name in *Through the Dragon's Eye*. The children took it in turns to take Gorwen home for the evening together with a special exercise book in which they had to write about what they and Gorwen had done together.

It was Androulla's turn today. She stepped up proudly to read from the exercise book her funny account of taking Gorwen with her to her swimming lesson.

> My mum asked Gorwen if he could swim and he said "No" so he had to wait in the car because we were scared he might drown. When we went home, my dad wanted to hug him and Gorwen blew fire and burnt his eyebrows off! Then we watched TV.

The children all laughed appreciatively.

"Poor Dad," commented Mrs Campbell with a twinkle in her eye. "It can't have been very nice having his eyebrows burnt off."

Androulla stood a little awkwardly fiddling with her skirt, biting her lip and unable to think of a smart reply. Just for a moment, perhaps she was thinking too literally about what she had written wondering whether she had really done some harm through her story. A seven-year-old's grasp of the difference between reality and fantasy can still be blurred at times. But Sara, Androulla's friend, chipped in helpfully with "They probably grew back when they were watching TV." Again the children laughed in approval at this suggestion.

What the children all recognized and enjoyed was that Gorwen's daily excursions to their homes and the resulting diary to which they all contributed was a kind of group fantasy which Mrs Campbell presided over. Gorwen belonged to them all, helping them to feel that they were part of a kind of family with a wayward younger sibling whom they cared for together. The exercise allowed them to use their imagination while at the same time encouraging them to represent the fantasy in writing practice. The children were able to give expression to their own fierce, fiery or nervous feelings in a harmless way by ascribing them to Gorwen and thereby exploring them at a safe distance. For those children in the class who were generally concerned to be seen as meek and good, it was refreshing to find a way to express a little fiery assertiveness and have such feelings accepted and contained within the group. At a more straightforward level, the Gorwen toy made for a wonderful home–school link. Parents were invited to help with the diary and enter into the spirit of the imaginative task. During other visits home, Gorwen had sampled exotic cuisine, played football, met childminders and grandparents, been to parties, mosques and churches and had generally broadened his horizons. His adventures were available for the children to read and share in the book corner, and it was a very well-thumbed volume.

Concentrating in class

Six- and seven-year-olds often find it quite a challenge to stay focused and maintain attention for long. The need to concentrate for a whole school day presents a big challenge to their maturity, and there is marked variation between individual children in their ability to persevere in the face of diffi-culty. Sometimes children may not be in the mood to work and become embroiled in some matter which is decidedly off-task, while, for others, it is too hard for them to hold on to a set of instructions. Good teachers put a great deal of effort into engaging their class in discussion, eliciting children's co-operation and making lessons as interesting as they can, but when all is said and done, daily practice of basic skills is the bread and butter of the school day and it simply has to be swallowed. The following example gives a flavour of the amount of effort that both children and teachers put in to the most ordinary of lessons. The challenge for the teacher or the classroom helper is to help individual children to see the task through to completion. Or, to put it another way, to enable them to concentrate sufficiently to overcome the allure of distractions.

The literacy task for this particular day in Mrs Campbell's class was to write about the reception class concert which these bigger, six- to seven-year-old children had been invited to watch the previous day. First, the teacher made sure that every pair of eyes was looking in her direction. She encouraged the children not only to comment on what they had seen but also to express an opinion about it. She tried to help them to think about what it felt like for the five-year-old reception children to perform in front of all those parents and older children, and what a lot of hard work the children and teachers had put in to choosing the music and making the costumes. They also discussed why it would have been unkind to laugh at the little girl who tripped onstage. With all this in mind, the children were to write an account of the concert, saying what they saw, what they liked and what they thought about it. There was a lot for the children to think about. The worksheets were given out and the children were asked to disperse to their tables.

A parent helper, Mrs Brown, had come in to the class to help that day and was asked to sit with a group of six children, three boys and three girls. The three girls were very interested in this new adult and were more enthusiastic about the possibility of getting to know her than in getting on with the writing task. Valerie liked her earrings. Mina wanted to tell her that she had a sore throat this morning and that her dad had given her a throat lozenge. To begin with, only Carl was able to get on in a straightforward way, while the others took a long time to gather themselves together. Valerie was very chatty and preoccupied with the pencils and whether she should sharpen them. Jack swung on his chair, made jokes, dropped his pencil and scrabbled around on the floor to find it. Anna simply looked blank and seemed genuinely to have retained nothing from the class discussion. After a moment or so Mina breathed a great sigh and made a start in spite of her sore throat, and Valerie settled down to work once her pencil had been sharpened, but they seemed able to do so only when they were confident they had Mrs Brown's attention. Gary pressed very hard with his pencil, was unhappy with the result and proceeded to rub it out, leaving a discouraging smudge on his clean worksheet. The whole table needed a great deal of prompting and encouragement. Six pupils seemed to Mrs Brown to be a very large group of children to support.

Some 15 minutes later, Mrs Brown's group was much more on track, but the minutes seemed to be ticking away very slowly. Carl had shown initiative in deciding to use a dictionary and had finished. Gary had managed one sentence in which there were many letter reversals and rubbings out, but he was trying hard to do what he thought was expected of him. Valerie had steamed ahead after a slow start. She seemed buoyed up by the helper's praise and interest in her, and she seemed to be almost understudying how this new grown-up was interacting with the group. In fact, it was Valerie's idea that Mrs Brown write some words on the blackboard so that everyone could spell them without having to keep asking. "Respectful" was the word she asked for. By contrast, Mina was finding it hard to stick with her writing. Instead she complained, "Anna's copying me, Miss. Tell her, Miss," and suddenly, the whole group were interested in how Mrs Brown would resolve the issue. Thinking quickly, Mrs Brown suggested to them that probably Anna wanted to share ideas rather than copy. That was OK, wasn't it? This seemed to satisfy Mina, who now managed to stay more focused, but before too long, Gary needed to go to the toilet, and strangely, once he had been given permission, Anna needed to go too.

In fact, by the end of the lesson time, the atmosphere had changed on Mrs Brown's table. Some definite headway had been made by each pupil but not without a great deal of adult input. Mrs Brown wondered how on earth the teacher managed when there were no parent helpers available. The children all seemed quite animated as they put their work away and prepared to go out to play. Mrs Brown, on the other hand, was exhausted.

4

Making Friends

How reassuring it is to find others who are like ourselves. Human beings are social creatures, and our six- and seven-year-olds are now grappling with the complicated business of making friends with other children. Now that they are spending more time away from their families, their peer group is becoming more influential in defining who they are. So it is that in a child's mind, "Who am I like?" is close to the question of "Who do I like?" In other words, children are looking for acceptance of themselves when they are seeking out friends. They need to check out their emerging identities with reference to other children. Popular children tend to be those who are self-assured, attractive and clever or have other desirable characteristics, and this can be damaging to children who feel they lack these qualities. At this age, friendships are likely to have their ups and downs. In fact adult attention and mediation are still needed by most six- and seven-year-olds to help them to develop satisfying ways of relating to each other. It will take them a long time to achieve a more mature basis for friendship based on give and take, empathy and respect for differences, but in the meantime it is helpful to have plenty of opportunities for practice.

Circle time

Schools make an active contribution to developing the social skills which children will need in order to get along with each other. Circle time aims to offer children greater understanding of social relationships and some simple strategies for managing conflict. Family life offers rich opportunities to learn about such matters as "give and take", sharing and respect for others, but, as we have seen in earlier chapters, a capacity to understand other people's points of view, to empathize with them, is something which is only just beginning to emerge at this age.

Many of the upsetting interactions between children at school come down to a lack of social understanding based on inexperience. Anyone who is familiar with children will know that they are very preoccupied with who is or is not their friend. Others' needs for personal space (in a physical sense) and for considerate treatment (in a moral sense) are very important foundations of citizenship which will take many years to acquire, but it is certainly not too early to make a start in actively promoting principles of cooperative living. Circle time allows children to focus their attention on matters which have, traditionally, been felt to be peripheral, or worse, an interference, in the school syllabus. Thankfully, modern schools recognize that they succeed when they are educating the whole child, and that children learn best from their experience and through example. So, the provision of a special space in the school day for thoughtful discussion of social matters helps children to feel that their everyday concerns are taken seriously.

It happened that one afternoon, just before the circle time session, some members of Mrs Campbell's class came in from playtime in tears. On exploration, it seemed there had been a minor altercation as the children were lining up to come in. Anna and James had a bruised leg and a bumped head between them, and they both blamed a third child for pushing as they were lining up to come in. Mrs Campbell took a few minutes to let the children involved tell her their different versions of what had happened, and dealt with it in a warm but matter of fact way. The distress was soon defused, but the incident led nicely into the topic for the circle time session, which was about "Saying sorry".

The children sat in a circle while their teacher asked them why they thought it was important to say "Sorry". The answers were sometimes a little obscure. "If you don't say sorry they will tell the teacher" was one suggestion. Many answers followed the previous idea but some expanded it. "If you do something to your friend, yeah, and you hurt their feelings – um, then they will tell of you and they won't be your friend." Mrs Campbell picked up on the new idea. "So, if you want to be friends it's a good idea if you say sorry." Using the recent incident in the playground as a starting point, she encouraged the children to think about how it feels to be pushed or hurt. She also helped them to think about the other point of view; what might it feel like to be shouted at for something you have done by accident? Some more complex questions arose. If you have done something to hurt another child on purpose, is simply saying "Sorry" enough to settle matters?

The lesson continued with the children being asked to talk to the child next to them about times when they have said "Sorry". They were instructed to take turns with the listening and the talking. The exercise seemed to capture the children's interest, and the classroom was buzzing with lively discussion. Later, Mrs Campbell asked pairs of children to make up little plays about what they had been discussing. The children took great pleasure in acting out scenes of various forms of unkindness: taking another's sweets, treading on toes and name-calling. All of this seemed familiar to them. The saying "Sorry" part of the lesson was almost incidental, almost an anti-climax, in fact. The children recognized that saying "Sorry" could be a useful formula for calming things down, but a sense of regret seemed some way off. This is hardly surprising. As adults we know that there can be world of difference between saying "Sorry" and really feeling remorse. Our adult wish for children to be sorry for their misdemeanours is often premature. An interesting question for this class of seven-year-olds might have been: "Have you ever said 'Sorry' and not really meant it?" but this was beyond the scope of the lesson. For now the children were learning that it is good to listen respectfully to the views of others, and helpful to let go of minor grievances, and these important lessons are important foundations of friendship.

In the playground

Freed from the demands of formal lessons, the school playground is a place to get rid of tension and just do what you like. By now the playground is a more familiar environment and if children have felt supported within the classroom, they will go out to play in anticipation of a safe interlude in which to let off steam with their friends. They are still under adult supervision and there is someone to turn to if things go wrong. Teachers and helpers on playground duty are important reference points and magnets for children looking for arbitration in minor disputes. Playground helpers are often shadowed by a following of friendly, chatty girls eager to make the most of a conversation with an interested adult. These adults also offer a sort of mobile paramedic service, giving judgements on the seriousness or otherwise of grazed knees, bumped heads and tummy aches. Six- and seven-year-olds know the routine and the playground is generally less daunting than it appeared when school was new to them.

This is certainly not to say that the playground is stress free. In the mêlée there are lots of parallel games going on with children drifting in and out of them. Social hierarchies are being established and challenged, best friends are tempted towards disloyalty with others and the sheer volume of noisy, running, excited children makes it a treacherous place for those who fail to look where they are going.

Some children come together to play imaginative games where each child is working out fantasies of his or her own in ways which trigger an interest in others. In this way imaginative games with a storyline sometimes emerge. Mina was noisily shouting instructions to Alison and Molly to steer a course to Mars. She was the leader in this game, and yelled that she was Supergirl going to save the planets. Two other girls tapped excitedly on the wall where their imaginary computers were located, and then, together with some other girls, they grappled fearlessly against imaginary aliens in a confused, raucous way amid many echoed shouts of "Supergirl to the rescue!" and a great deal of giggling. This was clearly a game for girls only and perhaps part of the fun of it was to exclude the boys.

Some playground games have survived in various forms from generation to generation. "Sticky Toffee" and its variations are popular, and this may be because they evoke the themes of a wish for greater independence set against an opposite current of wishing to be remembered, found and reclaimed. In this respect they invoke the relationship with the parents, to which children are linked by a sort of metaphorical elastic. Children of this age are pulling away from parents into the wider world but also enjoy a certain amount of being pulled back. In the game a child is chosen to do the chasing. The other children have to hold on to his or her fingers and thumbs, leading to a natural limit on the number of children who can play. The chaser shouts "Sticky Toffee" and the children scatter to avoid being caught. If a child is caught, he or she has to stand still with arms outstretched waiting to be freed by a child who has evaded capture. The last person is the winner and becomes the chaser next time. Rules are important to children and cheating can lead to quarrels and exclusion. Clapping games follow different sorts of rules and call for coordination, rote learning and pairing. These games seem to explore the idea of linking and separating and of being in synchrony with your friend. All of these games provide opportunities to explore a developing sense of identity and togetherness.

In the midst of all this thronging activity there will always be some children who find it difficult to join in. They may be missing home or lack the maturity, confidence or social skills to play cooperatively. Most children will have days when they feel like an outsider, but this will be more pronounced if they have worries which are related to life at home. On the other hand, some children's personalities may simply incline them towards more private, imaginative play. Such children may prefer to keep to the periphery of more exuberant activities and simply watch. It is not necessarily a problem if some children choose to keep themselves to themselves at playtime. A brief adult intervention can often encourage a shy child to try out joining in.

Androulla had been standing alone looking rather wistful, and was pleased when a passing playground helper approached her and said, "Hello". It turned out that Androulla was feeling sad because her best friend would not play with her. She was glad of the helper's interest and was keen to talk to her. In confidential tones, Androulla asked whether the helper would like to meet "Tweetie", and she showed her that she had a tiny blue plastic bird in her pocket. Tweetie was from her Snow White House (a toy from home) which was clearly very precious to her. Encouraged to go on, Androulla continued that when she is lonely she makes up songs about birds and flowers, which she sings to herself and to Tweetie. The helper was offered the little blue bird to hold and to examine, and their discussion continued until another girl from the same class wandered up. Androulla had been wondering whether Tweetie was a boy because he was blue and had short hair but the new girl was more pragmatic. Pointing to the little hole where Tweetie had been attached to the Snow White House she commented, "He must be a girl if that's his bum!" This comment seemed to have the effect of bringing Androulla back rather sharply into the playground world. The girls exchanged a few conspiratorial giggles, before wandering off arm in arm out of the helper's orbit.

Although Androulla was generally mature and competent in the classroom, she could feel a little lost in the playground, and used Tweetie rather like a three-year-old might use a teddy bear to keep a symbolic link with home, and more comforting feelings. Fortunately, the friendly interest of the playground helper helped her to feel more confident, so that when another girl came along she could engage with her more readily.

Gender identity

Children at this age are consolidating their identity and from a seven-year-old's point of view, gender is often the most significant dimension of self-definition. It is quite noticeable that the playground is beginning to divide into gender groupings. Left to choose their companions, six- and seven-year-olds are showing a marked preference for members of their own gender. If they are asked who they would like to come round to their home or who they would like to invite to their party, the chances are that boys will choose boys and girls will choose girls. Girls seem to have fewer friends but their relationships are more intense, while boys favour larger groupings.

Boys are coming to terms with what it means to be male, and this can be confusing in part. Passionate attachments to their mothers were more acceptable to their little boy selves, but these now become submerged beneath a preference for the company of their male friends. In this way boys are exploring what it means to have more independence and to be more like their dads or other role models. Not all boys are active and sporty but many take to active team games at this age, like ducks to water. Football, in particular, is a pastime which begins to appeal to large numbers of seven-year-old boys. There are different aspects of this. First, there is the game to be played which involves learning the rules and new physical skills. Second, there is the appeal of the professional sport to learn about, becoming a supporter of a particular team according to Dad's or other family members' affiliations. Third, there are many other football-related activities, such as computer games, sticker collections and table football. But perhaps above all, football provides a focus for the energy and desire to play with a group of friends and to have a defined sense of the "other side".

Playing football provides opportunities to get alongside other boys in a group setting which is bound together by the sorts of rules and hierarchies which seven-year-old boys like. The discipline required appeals to children's wish for orderliness and structure, which is so characteristic of this age group. However, the rules are complicated for six- and seven-year-olds to grasp at first, so there may be more of an interest in donning the kit and playing at being the famous footballer you most admire from the team that your dad supports. Running around and expending energy in a passionate way adds to the attraction of the game. All you need is a football and a decent sized area to play in. There is also the possibility of expending a lot of pent-up competitiveness and aggression and tempering this with the necessary cooperation and discipline required for a good game.

One frosty, late December morning a group of five six-year-olds had arranged to meet up at the local recreation ground together with three dads and two mums. Resplendent in their new football kits which Father Christmas had thoughtfully brought them, the boys were keen to act their parts. Ryan was among their number, sporting a Tottenham kit and the name Mendes with the number 8 on the back. The fun appeared to be in pretending to be a famous footballer while also learning some skills. "I'm Shearer!" shouted Joe to his father after a particularly satisfying muddy slide tackle. Keith took a tumble over Joe's outstretched leg and choked back a few tears. "Penalty!" shouted Joe's father, who was also the referee. Ryan was notable for keeping out of the fray. His mother noticed that he was particularly anxious not to dirty his new kit, although he gave the ball a good whack when it came in his direction. After a few minutes a minor scuffle broke out over possession of the ball. Joe's dad seemed to know instinctively how to defuse this: "Offside!" he shouted, catching the boys' eyes to make them move apart. The two mums chuckled to themselves about how useful it was to invoke the rules of football: far more effective than telling them to stop squabbling. There was a discipline here that all the boys were noticeably keen to respond to. The game continued until the dads were exhausted. Only then did Ryan seem to notice that his mum was there. "Did you bring me a drink?" he demanded, red faced. Ryan's mum knew with a certain poignancy that the drink would have to do as an expression of her pride in him. The cuddle that she felt like offering would not be acceptable in this manly context.

Girls' friendships tend to be more intense than those of boys and often rather more volatile. We have already seen how disoriented Androulla felt when her best friend would not play with her. Girls like doing things together, sharing secrets, playing more imaginative, pretend games and chatting together about all sorts of things. Fallings out resulting from covert rivalries and sensitive feelings are not uncommon. Perhaps it is because females tend to be more fine-tuned to personal feelings that their explorations of friendship are more fraught.

Some of the differences between groups of boys and girls can be exaggerated by six- and seven-year-olds, who may wish to make more of a split between themselves and those "others". One mother ran a "Rainbows" group (part of the scouting movement) for six- to seven-year-old girls. She noticed that the girls loved to absorb themselves in arts and crafts, drawing and tabletop games. Meanwhile, her husband ran a parallel group of "Beavers" at the Scout hut next door. His group were noisier, more physically active, and more of a challenge to manage in a group context. At the end of term they arranged for a joint get-together to be hosted by the Rainbows, who dutifully set out the drinks and biscuits ready for their guests. But the first boy to arrive was overwhelmed with embarrassment and revulsion. Flushing bright red he complained loudly, "I can't go in there, it's full of girls! Where are the other boys?" The other boys, it seemed, had assembled next door and felt able to face the girls only when there was safety in numbers.

Playing games and collecting things

Toys and games often help cement friendly contact between children at this age. The simplest of toys will generally do to fuel children's natural tendency to play creatively using their imagination. Playing and drawing are very important ways in which children represent their thoughts and feelings. In fact it could be argued that children are doing as much work through their play as they are in their more formal lessons, as it provides space for them to digest their emotional experience. Accordingly, children who do not play at all are rightly cause for concern. They may be too inhibited or troubled and may need specialist help to unblock what is usually a natural tendency.

Friendships between children are forged through shared interests expressed in play. Nowadays, children are subject to a great deal of targeted marketing through the media, and they also influence each other in involvement with the latest fads and crazes. When certain toys become a "must-have", we can assume that clever toy designers have tapped into something which resonates with children's own preoccupations. A look at the sorts of toys children choose gives clues about these.

Children of this age love collecting things. Whether the collection is of conkers, dolls, stickers, Power Rangers or Yu-Gi-Oh! cards, to name but a few possibilities, the point seems to be to amass a stockpile. The collection may represent a wish to have powerful resources. Children are not very clear at this age what it is that distinguishes adults' capacities from their own. They may feel that having a lot of something confers potency, thus helping them to feel that they have the resources to manage in a difficult and competitive world. Swapping with friends from their collection is a way of establishing commerce or give and take in its broader sense. "What do you have to offer me and what can I offer in exchange?" is a basis for a certain kind of cooperation.

Dolls have long been a favourite toy, usually for girls. The appeal may be at least in part about images of idealized womanhood. Baby dolls permit expression of maternal feelings, but also popular is a different kind of doll. Bratz™ dolls promote a feisty, teenager, glamorous, rock star image as desirable to six- and seven-year-old girls.

Board games promote the possibility of competing safely and according to agreed rules. These games are a good way to mobilize aggressive competitive urges without doing harm. At this age, however, children can be bad losers and parents often find themselves bending the rules a little to allow a child who is easily discouraged to have an experience of winning.

Children also like to make up their own games with rules. When Henry, a boy in the same class, came to Rashid's house for tea, they made up a game all about the names of children in their class. Henry and Rashid were on one team, since they were in the same class, playing against Rashid's sister, who was from a different class and had a different set of names to draw on. Rashid's mum was the referee and had to say a letter of the alphabet. The first child to say the name of someone in their class whose name began with that letter got a point. This was a rather touching way of keeping the whole class in mind, remembering them all as though part of a club. Six- and seven-year-olds can be very inventive, constructing games with rules out of almost anything, and pitting their wits against each other to score points.

Differences

There are many thought-provoking books for children exploring the theme of friendship, and one of these is *Willy and Hugh* by Anthony Browne. The story is about the blossoming of an unlikely friendship between two very different characters. In the story the two quite literally bump into each other. The smaller one, Willy, is more used to being picked on unfairly, and is amazed when the hefty Hugh apologizes to him. Willy apologizes too, and this leads on to friendship. The new friends discover that they have complementary strengths and can help each other. Hugh is good at chasing away the bullies who bother Willy, but Willy turns out to be the more level headed of the two and helps Hugh when he is terrified of a tiny spider. The story challenges in an amusing way the idea that it is best to seek out friends among those similar to oneself.

Children are learning about differences of race, colour, religion and language in their encounters with other children around them. Their feelings about others who are different from them is influenced by internal factors, but the attitudes encouraged at school play a significant part. Singing together at assembly time offers a medium through which children of this age can express their characteristic sense of wonder. Some songs also give voice to the hopes of the adult world. The lyrics of these two songs are particularly evocative:

Every colour under the sun

My hair's black and your hair's yellow –
My eyes are green and yours are blue.
There's no-one on earth who's quite like me
There's no-one who's quite like you.
And if you want to paint a picture of everyone
You'll need every colour under the sun.

From Every Colour Under the Sun. *Reproduced with*
permission from Ward Lock Educational Ltd.

Live it, love it

Our families come from many lands
From countries far and wide.
We speak in different languages
In which we all take pride.
In spite of all our differences
Which cannot be denied
You find so much in common if you look deep down inside.

Peter Gordon (2000). Reproduced
with permission (unpublished).

Learning to negotiate a social life is a complex business, and one of the most important things children are learning at this age. A friendly home life is likely to encourage a friendly disposition, and schools too are now actively teaching aspects of social understanding, but in the end children have to find their own ways to negotiate friendships. Although a child's friendship group will shift and change over time, the lessons learned now about group life and companionship are laying the foundations of successful grown-up life.

5

Reading for Meaning

For many parents, learning to read is one of the most important yardsticks for measuring learning at age seven. A capacity to read and to enjoy books is enormously enriching, opening up a world of possibilities for exploring knowledge of all kinds. An emotional readiness to learn to read comes when children feel secure enough to struggle with the difficulties involved. Children will have been helped to develop pre-reading skills through sorting activities and a range of opportunities to gain experience of associating letters and sounds. They will have been taught to recognize the shape of some of the more commonly occurring words and they will now be learning ways to combine cues from grammar, phonics and context, together with information from illustrations, to extend their level of reading skill. But the technical aspects of learning to read are secondary to the more holistic idea of reading for meaning, and this begins with the everyday experiences of family life. Modern educational practice recognizes that parents are the first teachers and that reading is most successfully learned through a collaborative approach between home and school.

Reading readiness

Although this may not be obvious, the foundations of reading are there in parental interactions with children from the very start of life. As mother talks and sings to them, babies begin to learn about the rhythms and cadences of spoken language. Soothed by Mother's voice, babies begin to associate language with feelings of comfort. As babies grow into toddlers, sharing warm interactions around nursery rhymes, stories and picture books gives them a sense of the value of listening and communicating with others.

Children become interested in understanding and making themselves understood if they have been listened to, thought about and communicated with in the day-to-day activities which parents initiate and maintain over time.

When children see their parents reading newspapers or magazines or working on a computer, or observe an older sibling doing homework, they are noticing that these activities are part of family culture in the broader sense and therefore an important part of their own potential identity. A wish to be like a parent leads to a curiosity about what it is that grown-ups like to do, and thus to becoming interested in sharing in reading-related activities. Parental support and encouragement are very important, and any opportunity to sit together quietly to share books and all sorts of print will feed children's natural enthusiasm to get to know both the world around them and the inner world of imagination. Making visits to the library a regular treat and choosing books as birthday presents also contribute to the idea that reading is special and fun.

Where English is the second language in a family, communication in English will, understandably, be hard for a child at first, but schools try to develop good home–school links before formal schooling begins, in order to find out more about the ways in which cultural patterns and mother tongue shape approaches to literacy. "Story sacks" are one example of a resource parents can use to construct narratives with their pre-school child. The sacks contain colourful objects and pictures which can be arranged into patterns to make up a story, together with simple books which depict the story as it has been constructed between parent and child. Some books for children are now available in two languages and scripts so that young children gain enriched experiences with written language. Such books are especially helpful for bilingual children, but all children benefit from learning that language can take many forms.

There are many pathways towards learning to read. Not all children go through the same stages and some may not use the same strategies as other children. It is rather like learning to walk. Many babies learn to crawl first, but some bypass this phase. Some babies learn a sort of bottom shuffle or a rolling technique for beginning to move around, but they all find ways to pull themselves upright in the end, and eventually launch off into their first steps. Similarly, in learning to read, children tend to get there in the end although they may learn in different ways and at very different paces. Although this is not a book about learning to read as such, it is worth exploring the relationships that underlie this big step in childhood.

As children are read to and share stories with a parent or teacher, they are entering into a more thoughtful, intimate relationship in which ideas can be explored. Children are getting to know the qualities of that other person, but they are still a long way from being able to do what the admired adults can do. There will be quite a gap in sophistication between stories which children enjoy when read to them and those that they can read by themselves. They need experience of both. An awareness of this disparity can be hard for a child to manage. In order to learn you need to be able to tolerate the fact that there are things that you do not already know, you need to put up with uncertainty and to bear frustration and disappointment when things go wrong. Keeping alive hopefulness in the face of failure is one of the hardest things for any learner. And this is so for adults as well as children. It can come as a shock to some children that learning does not happen magically and they need a good store of courage, determination and resilience in order to persevere. This comes from the experiences of being loved and valued. As we have seen in previous chapters, a certain amount of aggression, rivalry and competitiveness are helpful qualities of personality which propel a child onward when faced with difficulties, but if these characteristics are excessive they can interfere with a capacity to learn. Children also need to be able to continue to use the adults as supportive guides in their quest for understanding.

Putting the pieces together

Schools teach reading to six- and seven-year-old children by incorporating a number of strategies which includes developing a sense of belonging for all pupils and creating a warm, safe atmosphere in the classroom, so that taking risks with learning is more manageable. Classrooms for children of this age usually have a cosy inviting book corner with many picture books, and maybe also some examples of the children's own writing available to be read, like the Gorwen stories mentioned earlier. Their teachers usually try to make an arrangement for hearing individual children read at least once weekly, and they try to make this a special time for a more personal interaction with each child. Teachers also send reading books home regularly and encourage parents to take an active partnership with school in providing a quiet time for regular reading with their child. One-to-one attention with an adult is important in developing a child's confidence and sense of security, but group reading, and story time, where children sit together on the carpet to be read to by the teacher, are also key components of a classroom environment geared to promoting reading.

Through the Dragon's Eye

Many schools in the UK supplement their approach to teaching reading and literacy with a BBC *Look and Read* programme, where an exciting story in ten episodes provides an imaginative basis for project work over a whole term. The programmes are interspersed with little detours into word exercises set to music, rather as a conventional television programme might be punctuated by commercial breaks. At a less obvious level, the story introduces and addresses some of the difficulties and dilemmas that children face in learning to read. This symbolic content of the teaching aid is of particular interest to us here.

In Mrs Campbell's class, episodes of *Through the Dragon's Eye* were eagerly anticipated by the children. The characters became part of the classroom culture. In the story, the heroes are three children – Jenny, Scott and Amanda. They are a mixed group of children with different strengths and weaknesses to their personalities. The audience of six- to seven-year-olds can readily identify themselves with at least one of the characters. The children in the story have been painting a mural on the school playground wall under the supervision of their teacher. When Amanda makes the painting look more alive by painting in the dragon's eye, it comes to life and calls them into the painting, which is transformed into the magical land of Pelamar. Gorwen, the dragon, is their guide. He tells them that Pelamar is dying. The children's help is urgently needed because they can read, whereas he and the creatures of Pelamar cannot. The Veetacore (a sort of magical generator comprised of glowing blocks) has exploded, and three "veetons" (or components) are missing. The Veetacore is the life force of Pelamar, and it is looked after by the "Keepers", who have an ancient book to tell them how to look after it. Unfortunately, the Keepers have neglected their duties and have forgotten how to read. Worse than this, they have been doing their best to disguise this, and are at first resistant to accepting help from Gorwen and the children. With Gorwen's help, the children embark on a quest to save Pelamar by finding the missing veetons and putting the Veetacore back together again.

The story, thus, is an extended metaphor about overcoming obstacles to learning. Jenny, who freely admits that she is not a good reader, struggles to read a key passage in the book of the Veetacore: "The veetons, which have no power on their own, are related to and dependent upon one another."

Jenny mulls this over in her mind. Then she works it out: "I know, it's like a family. They fit together like a family."

Jenny discovers that she has a model of a family in her mind to help her struggle with fitting new ideas together. This is a source of inner courage when faced with difficulties. At another level, the veetons are like the letters of the alphabet, which fit together to make words and sentences in order to convey meaning. Learning to read, then, is a kind of puzzle in which the different strands of their experience come together in a symbolic way.

In *Through the Dragon's Eye* the main characters' quest to find the missing veetons leads them to encounter characters who obstruct them and make their task harder. These characters represent aspects of themselves which run counter to a wish to learn. In the story the Keepers seem to represent an attitude of mind which prefers not to know. They cannot see the point of learning to read, or rather, they have found reading too hard and have given up, preferring to believe that it does not matter. The children have to convince them by example that learning to read is worthwhile – it communicates vital information; it helps you to keep in touch.

The children also come across the Widgets. These are furry creatures who appear to be helpful and cute but turn out to be more interested in causing confusion and distraction. Perhaps they represent the mischievous, younger child aspects of six- and seven-year-olds, which can sabotage their more mature wish to struggle with the difficult aspects of learning. Maybe this is the lesson here for the pupils watching.

The story also contains a villain, as many children's stories do. Children of this age are very interested in the battle between "good" and "evil" as their sense of morality is developing. In the story, the evil Charn wants to destroy Pelamar. He is motivated by revenge and a greedy wish for power. The children in the story are frightened of Charn and have to find ways to outwit him. Back in the classroom the young viewers of the programme are sometimes a little frightened too, and so it is an important part of the project work that they are encouraged to talk about how the programme made them feel. A manageable amount of heightened feeling can be a great spur to creative work for children of this age, and this is often seen in the colourful, vibrant artwork produced and displayed in the classroom as part of the projects. Successful learning is often about overcoming fears, and children are gaining practice in this as they design and sew a "Charn" glove puppet or share a story about monsters, dragons or dangerous villains.

When stories capture the imagination of six- and seven-year-olds, as this one does, they become interested in writing, reading and chatting with their friends about the characters and the plot. Children of this age love to reconstruct stories that grown-ups have read to them and will often have a go at reading a book they know by following the pictures even if they cannot yet read the words. By contrast, when they are focusing hard on their technical skills it can be difficult to hold the thread of the story in mind and they can get either bored or frustrated. On the other hand, adults can do a great deal to help children with their reading when they encourage the idea that it is about something more than learning a technique and that books convey a world of meaning.

Difficulties with reading

Reading engages the whole personality and feelings such as worries about growing up play an important part in the process. Josh, for example, was big for his age but was actually one of the youngest in his class. He often had a sullen expression on his face and frequently regaled his teacher with tales of what the other children had done to him rather than paying attention to his own work. In fact he was often the one involved in classroom distractions. Josh did not look forward to reading with his teacher, reacting as though he would be criticized rather than encouraged. At a parents' evening his teacher discussed Josh's difficulties with his mother and father. His well-meaning parents admitted that they were finding it hard to manage Josh's moody behaviour at home. His mother compared him unfavourably with his three-year-old sister, Kim, who was felt to be easier and more affectionate. They said that Josh had been delightful, too, when he was a toddler, but now his father was concerned that if Josh did not start to apply himself to school work, it would be hard for him to get a good job in the future. His teacher noticed that Josh's parents spoke about him as though he was older than his six years, and Josh's large size may have added to the feeling that he should be taking more responsibility for himself.

In this discussion his parents began to see that Josh might be feeling under pressure. Learning to read had become a rather joyless activity linked in his mind to being pushed even further out of his parents' affections and into the grown-up world which he could not easily see the value of. Josh's parents were offered strategies to help them to encourage him more. He was also given some time in a less structured, small group setting at school. Once his difficulties had been recognized and understood, his reading and general demeanour rapidly improved.

There are some children who find it difficult to read because they mistrust authority. They want to be a success but are not easily able to bear being taught. Being "bossy" and telling the other children what to do rather than getting on with their own work is one way in which this sort of obstacle to learning is expressed. Suki was so fond of pretending to *be* the teacher that she did not listen properly to instructions. Her difficulties lay in her rivalry with the adults. She needed to "know" without having to be told, and found it very hard to bear being in her own seven-year-old skin. Her reading was rather slapdash and she could become very upset if corrected, responding as if cruelly cut down to size. She also found it difficult to make friends because of her overbearing manner. Her teacher discovered at a parents' evening that there were difficulties at home, with Suki being quite a handful for her rather worn-down single mother. Both Suki and her mother were offered some help at their local Child and Family Service and were both doing much better following a period of regular support. Not only did Suki become an avid reader but also she started to make friends.

At the other end of the spectrum it is hard for children to learn to read if they are very inhibited. Emma was a very shy six-year-old girl who had trouble learning the difference between the letters "b" and "d". This is actually a very common confusion at this age. Her teacher, Ms Tang, suggested a way to help her remember was to think of the word "bed". The "b" has to face forwards and the "d" backwards so that the shape of the word is like a bed. Emma looked confused, and when her teacher asked her what the matter was she mumbled, "I'm not allowed." She pointed to the "e" and said, "It's naughty." Ms Tang could not make sense of what Emma was trying to communicate to her, but she was attending a course on thinking about children's emotional development where she described this strange interaction to her colleagues. The group thought the "e" might stand for Emma, and that there was something on her mind about getting in the middle. The next time Ms Tang had an individual conversation with Emma, she asked her about this, and Emma was able to tell her that when she gets worried at night and tries to get into her parents' bed, they send her back to her room. This example shows that letters and words can often signify something quite personal and individual to children. They may become a way of giving expression to matters which already preoccupy them.

6

Confusions and Anxieties

Growing up is a confusing business. As we have seen, six- and seven-year-olds are fast developing skills and capacities that enable them to engage with the adult world in more subtle ways, but this comes at the cost of a loss of certainty. It is one of those paradoxes which we revisit throughout life, that the more we know, the more we realize what we do not know. Even more complicated, it can happen that the more we know, the more we would rather *not* know. This is particularly so for children at around seven, who are at the threshold of quantum leaps in understanding based on newly forged skills in literacy, social awareness and abstract thinking. They can feel competent and capable for more sustained periods of time but their immature personalities become easily overwhelmed. This fear of being overwhelmed by matters which are too complex for them sometimes leads to the formation of inhibitions and can surface in obscure anxieties which parents can find troubling. In this chapter we will take a look at some characteristic worries for children of this age group, and consider some typical parental preoccupations.

Feeling guilty

This is the age at which a guilty conscience can become more apparent as children become worried about the impact of their occasional wish to hurt or to deflect adult disapproval by a cover-up. One summer evening, Nadine, whom we heard about in Chapter 2, was having a water fight with her teenage stepsister. Out of the corner of her eye she spotted an unusual moth, which was camouflaged to look like a piece of twig. Her stepsister made a joke about it being an alien from outer space, and pretended to shoot it with her water pistol. Nadine screamed, taking her stepsister's words a bit too seriously. She opened fire with her own water pistol, hitting the moth with a torrent of water and making it fall over. But a moment later she was full of remorse. She tried to make amends by propping the moth up again with leaves, but this did not work. Overcome with emotion, Nadine rushed indoors to tell her mother what had happened. "Now the king of the moths will come and get me!" she added through frightened sobs.

Fortunately, her mother was able to take Nadine's worries seriously. They went together to examine the injured creature and found that it had, in fact, managed to right itself. Nadine was mightily relieved.

We cannot know for sure what was in Nadine's mind when she spoke about the king of the moths, but there was an idea of a vengeful figure who would punish her. Nadine's parents were not the vengeful sort, but the idea of something quite punitive was clearly a feature of the inner world of her imagination. Nadine was expressing what a guilty conscience feels like. Why she felt so guilty was not clear. Many children of this age are fascinated by "creepy crawlie" creatures, transforming them in their imaginations into "blood suckers", "slime monsters" and suchlike. Their own nastier feelings are disowned and located in the hapless life forms and can seem to come back at them as something threatening and scary. To some extent, children can quite enjoy frightening themselves with mini-monsters in an attempt to master fears about other unknowns. On this occasion, however, Nadine's worries about her destructiveness felt, momentarily, too much for her to manage. Nadine knew that her parents were thinking about having another baby. She was already quite jealous of her stepsister and the idea of another rival might, possibly, have been on her mind when she attacked the moth. Seemingly irrational anxieties like Nadine's are common in children of this age and can cause a lot of worry to them.

"Are Mum and Dad all right?"

This is not likely to be an anxiety which a child will articulate directly, but it is nonetheless likely to be around from time to time. As children become aware that their parents are not all-powerful they are more likely to be concerned about them, particularly if there are vulnerabilities in a parent that they are aware of. Single parents, those who are unsupported in other ways, or parents who are in conflict with one another may sometimes evoke concern or worry in a sensitive child. Temporary difficulties are a feature of everyday life and it does children no harm to observe their parents grappling with difficulties of various sorts as long as this is set in a context in which they basically feel loved and wanted. It is impossible to protect children completely from ordinary adversity. But children are very astute and notice when all is not well, so it is better when difficult circumstances can be acknowledged in an appropriate way.

"Who will I be like?"

Boys are now actively looking for male role models and thinking about their own maleness. What sort of man might they become in the future? Boys growing up without a father, for whatever reason, will be looking to their mother to check out their ideas about what maleness means. So it is particularly hard for boys if mothers who have a low opinion of their child's biological father pass this judgement on to him. The child may well wonder whether he is going to be like this denigrated man when he grows up. It is immensely helpful in such circumstances if there are other good father figures around, either within the family or as part of the mother's supportive network of friends. The same applies for girls, and for children of both genders living with single fathers. When children have to live in foster care or adoptive families, it is generally because there have been major difficulties in their families of origin, so that for them concerns about who they might be like, in future, may be all the more acute. Whether together or separate, present or absent, biological parents are very much part of any child's identity. Even if children do not know their absent parent, they will have thoughts and theories about them and it is nearly always helpful if their questions can be answered in a reasonably straightforward way without going into too much unnecessary detail. But it is just as important for parents to recognize that children are unique. Genetics do contribute to personality, but experiences of life count for more.

Sexual feelings

Seven-year-old Amy enjoyed playing on her own with her Barbie® dolls – dressing them, combing their hair, taking them on imaginary shopping trips and having tea parties. When her aunty bought her a male doll called Ken to add to her collection, Amy was unsure how to include the newcomer in her games. She had an idea that the male and female dolls might go to discos and kiss and do other things which she suspected went on between her parents at night-time. She decided to remove the doll's trousers to see what she could discover about these mysterious matters. To her disappointment, Ken was completely without genitals. Now Amy felt rather disgusted with Ken, who had seemed to invite exploration of matters she felt mixed up about. She decided to use the doll for a very different game. Wrapping him up tightly in a bandage, she decided he was to be an Egyptian mummy, such as she had been learning about at school. As she covered up the Ken doll, perhaps she wanted to cover over her sexual curiosity as well. Once thoroughly wrapped, Ken was consigned to a drawer and largely forgotten about, and the tea parties with her Barbies could resume undisturbed.

Amy, like many children of her age, was both fascinated and repelled by the whole area of matters sexual. She was particularly close to her mother and was rather jealous of the relationship between her parents, which excluded her and had led, somehow, to the birth of her younger sister. Although Amy was keen on watching TV programmes aimed at young adolescents, such as *Top of the Pops*, which involved a lot of provocative dancing and singing, she herself was going through a phase where she would wear only trousers and was no longer interested in the dresses and skirts she had loved to wear a year ago. Amy seemed to be trying to hold at bay her awareness that she was a long way from being sexually mature, and, like Ken, rather inadequately equipped to join in the world of adult sexuality. While being unable to deny her interest in the exciting private life of the adults, Amy was relieved to put aside her longing to be involved. In her game with the dolls she transformed her sexual interest into a school-related one. The Ancient Egyptians were from far away and long ago. For the moment at least, six- and seven-year-olds often try to put quite a distance between themselves and more passionate longings.

On the other hand, children are very interested in the relationships between their parents and between other couples. These relationships can be seen as very exciting and are played out in the playground in games like "Kiss-Chase", but children are also interested in the more tender, loving feelings which cement adult relationships, especially when they experience this at home. They themselves may develop attachments to a "sweetheart" in an earnest sort of way. These themes are explored in a delightful picture story-book for this age group entitled *Jennifer Jones Won't Leave Me Alone* by Frieda Wishinsky and Neal Layton. In the story a romance blossoms between two classmates in a rather touching way.

Toilet humour

Children can now take care of their personal hygiene to a greater extent. They are expected to be continent, both in a literal and a metaphorical sense. Eating is something which is sociable and public, whereas going to the toilet is something which is private and about which we hope to make as little fuss as possible. Children of this age tend to know the difference between what is socially acceptable and what could be described as being rude, but the latter holds a certain inevitable attraction to them. When we talk about a childish sense of humour, we usually mean the sort that refers to bodily functions. There are many popular TV programmes for children which tap in to this childhood fascination. *Get Your Own Back*, for example, is a UK quiz game where a child gets to interrogate the parent. If the parent answers the questions incorrectly she is good-humouredly lowered into a vat of "gunge", which is horribly evocative of sewage. Children can derive a feeling of potency through their private bodily functions, and they understand what embarrassment is. What fun to trick your granny into sitting on a "Whoopee Cushion" and making an embarrassing noise! But the humour here is at some level linked to anxiety. Children are often worried that they will make a mess or be exposed to ridicule. The incongruity of making Granny into the naughty one can be a way of dealing with anxieties at a distance by pushing them into someone else with a trick. Thankfully, grannies often have a sense of humour too and usually don't mind.

Monsters under the bed

Going to bed and falling asleep means letting go, trusting the adults to be in charge and relaxing body and mind. But if a child is stirred up with feelings for whatever reason, going to sleep, like any temporary separation, will require some preparation. It is quite usual for six- and seven-year-olds to develop rituals around bedtime to keep anxieties at bay. Ali required his dad to check under his bed for monsters each evening before he would get into bed. This had become a regular routine. Some children like to arrange the curtains in a particular way to have a regulated amount of light or darkness in their room. For others the way in which they are tucked in becomes important. One seven-year-old who had had a very troubled early life and was living in foster care insisted that at night he held on to one end of a long piece of string linking his bed to his foster mother in her bedroom. The idea was that he could pull on it to get her to come if he had bad dreams. Night-time is when worries can surface, particularly those linked to fears of loss or reprisals for bad thoughts or deeds.

A regular routine and a certain amount of bedtime ritual is helpful so that a child can wind down and prepare for sleep. A bedtime agreed well in advance can reduce arguments about parental arbitrariness. Showers or baths followed by tooth brushing are part of the ritual. Computer games, especially the exciting, competitive ones, tend to increase the level of a child's arousal and make getting to sleep more difficult. Reading stories together, or offering a story tape, are by contrast soothing and calming ways to prepare for sleep. It is often at bedtime that children may want to talk about things that are on their mind – issues about school, friends or more obscure mixtures of fantasy and reality like the example of Nadine and the king of the moths. A few minutes to listen respectfully to whatever it is that is concerning a child, even if the concern sounds rather ridiculous, goes a long way. As we have seen, children of this age are not always able to express their worries in a logical way. But delaying tactics at bedtime need to be borne in mind. Any child needs to know that parents can be firm but fair about actually taking their leave. Sometimes it is the parent's state of mind which a child is concerned about when it is time for "lights out" and indeed there are bound to be times when parents are feeling vulnerable. All the more reason, if possible, to demonstrate that one is there to look after the child and not have things the other way round.

Once a good routine is established, sleeping is not usually a problem. The odd nightmare is generally recognized by a child at this age for what it is – just a dream. Persistent nightmares and failure to sleep are rare, but if they continue beyond a short phase it may be advisable to seek help via your family doctor, who would be likely to refer on to a local Child and Family Consultation Service or a similar organization.

"It's not fair!"

Children tend to blame their parents for the ordinary frustrations of life and "It's not fair!" is a common complaint. But if we listen closely there may be more to this than just petulance. At around six or seven children are making some fairly indigestible discoveries about the world, and who, if not their parents, can be a sounding board to help them to bear some of these painful truths? If we can bear in mind that a child is really struggling with something difficult we are more likely to be understanding of a child's sense of injustice.

Primarily, children notice that they are not the same as their parents or older children. They have to learn to tolerate that they are relatively inexperienced. In reality older siblings can manage more than they can and this can be hard to bear. For example, on Mother's Day, Ryan's older brother and sister decided to take breakfast upstairs to their mother for a treat. Ryan wanted to make the toast and carry the tray but the older ones said he would probably burn himself on the toaster and spill the tea on the stairs. An angry argument ensued and their father had to intervene to keep the peace. "You never let me do anything!" Ryan protested. "It's not fair! Mum will like them best!" Ryan felt convinced that his mum would prefer his more mature siblings because they were more like adults in preparing breakfast. In truth, the older ones were a bit too ready to make Ryan feel redundant as a helper. His father managed to mollify him a little by suggesting he carry Mum's card to her, but Ryan was still rather out of sorts. It was only when Mum shared her toast with him that Ryan felt better. It may be that he was also relieved that the proper order of things had been restored. After all, it is the mothers who are supposed to feed the children and not the other way round. Like many six- and seven-year-olds Ryan wanted to be part of things in his family but the sense of potential unfairness was not far from the surface when differences between siblings were exposed.

At this age there are many inexplicable facts about life that may simply seem unfair. Children feel that it is unfair that people die. With an increased awareness of the passage of time comes the recognition that growing old also happens to those one loves. Children come to have a reasonable understanding that their parents and grandparents have a finite life expectancy which is different from their own. At a less exalted level, it can also feel unfair that children in the same class learn at different rates or that children in the same family have different bedtimes. Some families can afford a particularly desirable toy whereas another family cannot. The list of unfairnesses is potentially endless, and even so, we adults, with our greater knowledge of the wider world, know that our six- and seven-year-olds know little, as yet, of political injustice or social inequality.

The poignancy of children's complaints perhaps lies in their belief that things *should* be fair and that they have been robbed of something they were entitled to expect. This is all part of a wider realization, at this age, that much as we would like to settle things simply, with clear-cut rules, regulations and predictability, life can be perplexing. Parents cannot make the world fair but fair-mindedness in our interactions with our children helps them not to be too disappointed in the realization that it takes a long time to grow, to learn and to gain more understanding.

Some parental concerns

Food

Food is symbolic of the love and care parents offer a child. When the child was younger, feeding was much more under adult control, but is now rather less so. There are many concerns these days about the quality of school dinners, about TV advertising for fat, sugar and salt-laden foods during children's viewing times, and about peer pressure when it comes to eating. Obesity is a serious problem in many Western societies. What can a parent do to keep a child healthy? One important aspect to consider is children's difficulty in making choices. They tend to want to be like the others. Most school dinners offer "healthy" options but children may find it hard to choose them. Some parents get round this by sending a packed lunch. A child may prefer this for a while and then beg to revert to school dinners or vice versa, according to what his or her friends are having. It can also happen around this age that children may suddenly decide they no longer like broccoli, tomatoes or some other food which they had enjoyed before, and this can sometimes be tied up with struggles over authority. *Eat your Peas* by Kes Gray and Nick Sharratt is an amusing picture storybook about stubbornness in relation to food. In the story, a child's refusal to eat her peas on the grounds that she does not like them is met by her mum's offers of increasingly desperate (and funny) inducements to get her to eat them. The illustrations of Mum show her wearing earrings and a necklace which look like peas, suggesting that there is a sort of metaphor here for aspects of her mum's limit setting which the child finds "hard to swallow". In the story a friendly compromise is reached in the end, and the point is made that parents can get overly concerned to make children eat certain things. In fact, children's food fads generally shift over time, when the rest of the family are seen to enjoy their food and when mealtimes are not too stressful.

TV, computers and electronic games

There are some terrific TV programmes for children of this age and watching them can be a good way of winding down after a hard day at school. The key here is to try, if possible, to promote a sense of discrimination and to help children to make good use of the "off" button. Too much television leaves no time for other activities. It is certainly true that there are excellent computer games and Internet sites designed for children, which are fun, educational and help to improve skills. On the other hand, computer games, with their fast rewards and endless challenges, can prove overwhelming in large doses. One mother found that her seven-year-old son became irritable and bad tempered if he had more than a half-hour session on his GameBoy®. In short, active parental guidance is needed to help children to manage these media. Parents do need to be vigilant in these days of cable TV where among the large number of channels there is more likelihood of children coming across programmes which are too violent, scary or sexually explicit. The same is true of the Internet, where children find it all too easy to stumble across inappropriate material. Locks and filters on your computer are a very good idea.

Danger

Now that children are beginning to make more of a bid for independence, parents are likely to be concerned about how to keep them safe in a world which appears increasingly hazardous. Children of this age are now learning to cross the road with care but it is still difficult for them to judge the speed of oncoming traffic. Parents are often concerned about dangers of a more insidious kind and rightly warn their children about the importance of not accepting sweets or lifts from strangers. If children have had experience in an ordinary family context of their "No"s or other refusals being taken seriously, then by the age of six or seven they will be more confident about asserting their likes and dislikes in other contexts also. Similarly, children who are reasonably secure now know that close physical contact is appropriate within the family but not with comparative strangers. Whether or not there are more dangers to children than there used to be is hard to say, but there is certainly more awareness in society of potential dangers. Children who are forewarned in an appropriate way are likely to be safer.

Conclusion: Celebrating Achievement and Moving On

As the summer approaches the school year is drawing to a close, and this is a time for taking stock of gains and thinking about future directions. Children in England take national attainment tests at the start of the summer term, to check that they are reaching the standards expected for seven-year-olds. Although schools do their best to keep this testing low key, it is still a relief for all concerned when these have been completed and can be put to one side. Now it is the season for celebration of the year's achievements with end-of-year concerts, summer fêtes and parties.

The summer concert is a joyous occasion. So much planning and rehearsal go into these events with everyone – teachers, pupils and parent helpers – playing their part. Colourful costumes are created and dances are choreographed and put to music to produce a marvellously entertaining show. This is a chance for the children to shine and for the audience of parents, family and friends to experience a warm glow of pride in their child's performance. Photographs and home videos are eagerly captured, bearing witness to the fact that for both children and parents these are memorable moments to be treasured forever.

Mrs Campbell's class performed an adaptation of their favourite project and called it "Trouble in Pelamar Again". Their concert incorporated their favourite characters in a musical quest which took them to a rich range of locations in search of missing veetons. Androulla was part of a scene in a desert where they sang a song about riding on a camel. Gary and Mina had their chance next, as the action moved to the fictional land of Widge. Dressed in furry costumes as Widgets, they performed an acrobatic dance involving rolypoly moves to a cheeky, chattering musical accompaniment. Taking slow giant strides and dressed in silver, Valerie took part in a scene in space. Carl, meanwhile, concentrated hard on his task of playing percussion instruments right on cue. Ryan had been practising speaking loudly and clearly in order to deliver his contribution as narrator and this certainly paid off on the day. The whole performance came to a climax with a rousing chorus of "Climb Every Mountain" and the sea of earnest shining faces brought forth rapturous applause, with hardly a dry eye in the audience.

Once the excitement of the concert had subsided there was still time left for important work to ease the transition to the next year group. Seven-year-olds know that they will shortly be saying goodbye to their teacher and will be preparing for the real and imagined changes that the next school year may bring. In the UK, moving from being one of the oldest in the infant school to one of the youngest in the junior school can feel rather daunting. This is likely to mean some changes in teachers' expectations and perhaps some additional privileges. Many schools do their best to ease the transition in thoughtful ways. The children in Mrs Campbell's class each received a letter from a pupil in the class they would be moving to in the autumn, telling them about some ways in which the junior school is similar to and different from the infants. Ryan heard from a boy called Luke, who told him that they have a lunchtime club where they can learn to play chess, they are allowed to write in pen rather than pencil, and there is a brand new library. On the down side, however, there is more homework, you can get detention if you are really naughty and school starts five minutes earlier than in the infants. The message from Ryan's point of view was that they clearly mean business up there. The infants children wrote back politely, following discussion in their class group, saying what they were and were not looking forward to. They followed this up with a visit to their new classroom together with Mrs Campbell. In this and other ways the children were being prepared to move on, but for some it would still be a wrench to leave behind the security of the infants school and their kindly teacher, who never gave detentions.

In this book we have tried to open some new doors to enrich our under-standing of the world of six- and seven-year-olds. So it seems only fitting to give the last word to a seven-year-old. Ryan had been giving a lot of thought to his change of status over the school summer break. Asking his mother whether he could use her pen, he decided to write a story. Ryan was clearly thinking about incremental steps towards growing up and even, eventually, growing older when he wrote this story called "The Ladybird's Spots". This is what he wrote:

> Once there was a ladybird called Tom.
> He was a very nice ladybird.
> One day that ladybird went to his granddad.
> He told Tom that when he has one spot he will be able to jump.
> When he has two spots he will be able to swim.
> When he has three spots he will climb really high.
> When he has four spots he will be able to make things disappear and come back again in a different place.
> When he has five spots he will ride a bike with black spots on.
> When he has six spots he will be able to talk to humans.
> When he has seven spots he will be able to skip.
> When he has eight spots he will be able to survive for as long as possible.
> So Tom had a very nice life.
>
> THE END

And so it was that Ryan set the stage for moving on to eight, expressing the hope that the next years would offer him "a very nice life".

Further Reading

Bettelheim, B. (1982) *On Learning to Read: The Child's Fascination with Meaning*. London: Thames & Hudson.

Hindle, D. and Vaciago-Smith, M. (eds) (1999) *Personality Development: A Psychoanalytic Perspective*. London: Routledge.

McClellan, J. (2001) *A Parents' Guide to the Internet*. London: Atlantic (on behalf of Guardian Newspapers).

Salzberger-Wittenberg, I., Henry, G. and Osborne, E. (1983) *The Emotional Experience of Learning and Teaching*. London: Routledge & Kegan Paul.

Waddell, M. (1998) *Inside Lives: Psychoanalysis and the Development of the Personality*. Tavistock Clinic Series. London: Duckworth.

Winnicott, D. W. (1964) *The Child, the Family and the Outside World*. London: Penguin.

Storybooks referred to in this book

Browne, A. (1992) *Willy and Hugh*. London: Red Fox.

Gray, K. and Sharratt, N. (2001) *Eat your Peas*. London: Red Fox.

McKee, D. (1997) *Two Monsters*. London: Red Fox.

Mooney, B. (2003) *But You Promised!* London: Egmont (part of the "Kitty and Friends" series).

Northway, J. (1993) *Get Lost, Laura!* London: Scholastic.

Shields, C. D. and Meisel, P. (1997) *I Am Really a Princess*. London: Orchard.

Simon, F. (2005) *Horrid Henry's Big Bad Book*. London: Orion (latest of the "Horrid Henry" series).

Waddell, M. and Dale, P. (1991) *Once There Were Giants*. London: Walker.

Wishinsky, F. and Layton, N. (2004) *Jennifer Jones Won't Leave Me Alone*. London: Picture Corgi.

Helpful Organizations

British Broadcasting Corporation
PO Box 1922
Glasgow G2 3WT
Tel: 08700 100 222
www.bbc.co.uk/children
A useful hub for information, educational advice and games to play with children online

ChildLine
45 Folgate Street
London E1 6GL
Tel: 020 7650 3200
Helpline: 0800 1111 (for children and young people)
www.childline.org.uk
Confidential 24-hour helpline for children and young people

Exploring Parenthood
Latimer Education Centre
194 Freston Road
London W10 6TT
Tel: 020 8964 1827
Parents' Advice Line: 020 8960 1678
Advice on parenting problems from newborn to adult

Gingerbread Association for One Parent Families
7 Sovereign Close
London E1W 2HW
Tel: 020 7488 9300
Advice Line: 0800 018 4318 (Monday to Friday 9 a.m. to 5 p.m.)
www.gingerbread.org.uk
Support for single-parent families

Lifeline for Parents
101–103 Oldham Street
Manchester M41 LW
Tel: 0800 716 701 (helpline Monday to Thursday 5 p.m. to 9 p.m.)
Information and support for parents

National Literacy Trust
Swire House
59 Buckingham Gate
London SW1E 6AJ
Tel: 020 7828 2435
www.literacytrust.org.uk
Aiming to improve literacy by promoting the fun of learning and the importance of book choice

Parentline Plus (formerly National Stepfamily Association)
Tel: 0808 800 2222 (helpline 24 hours a day)
www.parentlineplus.org.uk
Information and support for parents

YoungMinds/National Association for Child and Family Mental Health
102–108 Clerkenwell Road
London EC1M 5SA
Tel: 020 7336 8445
Parents' Information Service: 0800 018 2138
www.youngminds.org.uk
Campaign to improve the mental health of children and young people

Index

relationships
    children's interest in 62
    in class 35
    with class teacher 18, 32–4
    with classmates 18–19
    friendships 41–5, 49–50
    with parents 27
    between siblings 26–7
rewards, in school 35
right and wrong 20
rivalry *see* competitiveness
rude humour 63

safety 67
schools
    behavioural management 35
    playgrounds 43–5, 62
    routines 34
    school life 31–9
    teaching of reading 53–4
self
    sense of 15, 18
    see also identity
setting limits 30
sexuality 61–2
Sharratt, N. 66
Shields, Carol Diggory 21
shyness 57
siblings, rivalry with 26–7
Simon, Francesca 26
single-parent families, role models 61
skills, learning 19
social education 41–3
songs 49–50
spoken language 16–17
sports (football) 46–7
'Sticky Toffee' game 44
stories, in learning to read 54–6
story sacks 52
summer concerts 69
swearing 16–17

talking with children 16–17, 41–3, 64
teachers, relationship with 18, 32–4
television 66, 67

telling tales 35
thinking, literal 21
thinking skills 13, 17–19
three-dimensional thinking 17
Through the Dragon's Eye 35–7, 54–5
time, understanding passage of 28, 65
toilet humour 63
tooth fairy 21–2
toys 48
transitions 24
truth, understanding about 20
Two Monsters 18

Wishinsky, F. 62
worries 59–67